Documentation: The Language of Nursing

ERMA COTY, MSN, RN

JEFF DAVIS, BSCS, RN

LISA ANGELL, BSN, RN

Cartoons by Erin Angell

Prentice Hall Health
Upper Saddle River, New Jersey 07458

Library of Congress Cataloging-in-Publication Data

Coty, Erma
    Documentation : the language of nursing / Erma Coty, Jeff Davis, Lisa Angell ;
cartoons by Erin Angell.
        p. ; cm.
    Includes bibliographical references and index.
    ISBN 0-8385-1723-4
    1. Nursing records—Programmed instruction. 2. Nursing records—Computer-assisted instruction. 3. Nursing—Terminol-
ogy—Programmed instruction. 4. Nursing—Terminology—Computer-assisted instruction. I. Davis, Jeff, 1957-II. Angell, Lisa.
III. Title.
    [DNLM: 1. Nursing Records—Programmed Instruction. 2. Nursing Records—Terminology—English. 3. Documentation—
Programmed Instruction. 4. Documentation—Terminology—English.
WY 18.2 C852d 1999]
RT50.C67 1999
610.73′01′4—dc21

                                                                                                    99-049884

Publisher: *Julie Alexander*
Editor-in-Chief: *Cheryl Mehalik*
Acquisitions Editor: *Nancy Anselment*
Editorial Assistant: *Beth Ann Romph*
Marketing Manager: *Kristin Walton*
Marketing Coordinator: *Cindy Frederick*
Director of Production and Manufacturing: *Bruce Johnson*
Managing Production Editor: *Patrick Walsh*
Senior Production Manager: *Ilene Sanford*
Production Liaison: *Cathy O'Connell*
Creative Director: *Marianne Frasco*
Cover Design: *Wanda España*
Composition: *Clarinda Company*
Project Management: *York Production Services*
Printing and Binding: *Banta Company—Menasha*

©2000 by Prentice-Hall, Inc.
Upper Saddle River, New Jersey 07458

ISBN 0-8385-1723-4

Prentice-Hall International (UK) Limited, *London*
Prentice-Hall of Australia Pty. Limited, *Sydney*
Prentice-Hall Canada Inc., *Toronto*
Prentice-Hall Hispanoamericana, S.A., *Mexico*
Prentice-Hall of India Private Limited, *New Delhi*
Prentice-Hall of Japan, Inc., *Tokyo*
Prentice-Hall (Singapore) Pte. Ltd.
Editora Prentice-Hall do Brasil, Ltda., *Rio de Janeiro*

Care has been taken to confirm the accuracy of information presented in this book. The editors, and the publisher, however, cannot accept any responsibility for errors or omissions or for consequences from application of the information in this book and
make no warranty, expressed or implied, with respect to its contents.

The authors and publishers have exerted every effort to ensure that drug selections and dosages set forth in this text are in
accord with current recommendations and practice at time of publication. However, in view of ongoing research, changes in
government regulations, and the constant flow of information relating to drug therapy and drug reactions, the reader is urged
to check the package inserts of all drugs for any change in indications of dosage and for added warnings and precautions. This
is particularly important when the recommended agent is a new and/or infrequently employed drug.

Dedication

To my dad, Andrew Parise, who always believed I would write, and to my husband, Doug, who with my children believes that I can do just about anything. ELC

For two nurses who embody our profession, my grandmother Mary Sarvela and my mother Monica Clark, both of whom devoted themselves to caring for their families as they cared for their patients. And to my wonderful daughter Erin who has unlimited patience and humor with her mom. LSA

To the many patients who, even in times of pain and distress, have managed to express their thanks. I am always amazed by this ability. JLD

Contents

Preface

When Erma, Lisa, and I first met to discuss the potential need for a book about the language of nursing, we knew that the topic was important. During our accumulation of a significant amount of experience in a variety of nursing disciplines, we had each learned that communication was a cornerstone of good patient care. We also knew that, like any technical discipline, nursing used language in a unique, uncommon way to establish and maintain that communication. Of course, the medical world possessed a vocabulary all its own, and nurses needed to understand and use that vocabulary. We concluded, however, that the language of nursing encompassed more than mastery of the medical jargon. In fact, we noted that a great many technical words were common to the layman, but had special meaning and intention when applied to nursing. We decided that to become good at speaking in "nurse," one had to practice using the language. Thus, we formulated the idea for an interactive tool that student nurses could use to exercise and drill. We came up with this interactive textbook and the accompanying computer application.

The overall design of the textbook and the computer program is that of flexibility and drill. The book is chronological in that basic concepts are introduced at the beginning, and the material progressively builds from there. However, the user need not walk through the text from front to back. The interactive exercises, especially, may be selected in any order, although they do increase in complexity as the book progresses. The computer application reflects this flexibility with its ability to jump to any exercise in any chapter.

There is an emphasis on repeated practice. Although this may at first sound tedious, we believe that the format of the text and exercises keep things moving. We use a variety of exercises to help prevent boredom without loss of consistency. Through practice, the student can see how words are used; we attempt to stimulate this throughout the textbook. Thus, it is our intent to expose the student to similar material more than once. In fact, we suggest that users may make several passes through the textbook, or at least repeat exercises in some of the chapters. The interactive computer program is especially conducive to this.

USE OF THE TEXT

A word list introduces most chapters. We recommend using this list as a drill by trying to assign both a common, layman's definition and then a technical, nursing definition to each word. As each chapter progresses, concepts are explained, with focus material emphasized or detailed in text boxes. After most concepts, at least one exercise is presented before moving on to a new idea. If an explanation in the text is not clear, just move on to the corresponding exercise. Go back to the explanation later. Repeat the exercise. Complexity of concepts and exercises increase as chapters progress.

USE OF THE COMPUTER APPLICATION

The interactive computer application, called **WorkBook,** is provided as an adjunct to the text material. By using it, the student can easily repeat exercises, as well as pick and choose those he or she may wish to focus upon. A short synopsis of each chapter is also readily available.

Most text chapters have an accompanying chapter in the WorkBook application, with exercises similar to those in the textbook. Some of the exercises in the text are not available for the computer, and others are adapted with changes. In most cases, this is because the exercise answers are in written narrative, and the complexity of checking correctness of such answers is beyond the scope of most computer programs.

In producing the interactive computer application, we assumed only a basic understanding of personal computers on the part of the user. If the reader can open an application in Microsoft Windows version 3.1 or later, she or he can use the WorkBook application. We have provided details on use of the application in Appendix C.

Our goal in the text and the computerized material is to provide an easy medium to practice the language of nursing. We hope that both students and practicing nurses find it to be light and entertaining, as well as beneficial.

Jeff Davis

Contributors

Cathy Glynn-Milley, RN, CRNO
Principal, Specialty Nursing Agency, Inc.
Santa Clara, California

Patricia M. Duca, BSN, RN
Santa Cruz, California

Joan E. MacKay, RNC
Principal, Specialty Nursing Agency, Inc.
Santa Clara, California

Frances Tso-Yee, RN, MSN, NPC
Adult Nurse Practitioner
Olive View–UCLA Medical Center
Los Angeles, California

Michael Linden McGannon, MD, FACEP
Watsonville, California

Acknowledgments

Many people have contributed to the evolution of this text from idea to reality: Kelly Radner, who suggested we write it and who put us in contact with Lauren Keller, who believed in the concept. We owe thanks to the student nurses of Cabrillo College in Aptos, California, particularly K. W., who was relentless in having me search for a text on charting. Thanks to all those who contributed to this project with wisdom, anecdotes, and good humor, and to Donna Duell, RN, who was supportive and encouraging throughout the process. And, a very special thank you to Dave Carroll, our editor and friend, who trusted that this unusual project was worthwhile and timely.

Personal thanks to Eunice Brown, RN, for her special insight, to Doug E. Coty for reality checks and for making sure the computer kept working, to Paul and Johnna Coty, and to Doug P. Coty, who contributed daily by keeping things in perspective.

Thanks to Mark Davis, Rich Turner, Kelly Mitter, and June Fallon for their support during the life span of this project.

Thanks to Erin Angell for her patience, good humor, and drawing skills. Thanks to Donald North for his interest and encouragement.

Bibliography

Bates, B. (1991). *A Guide to Physical Examination and History Taking* (5th ed.). Philadelphia: J. B. Lippincott.

Burrell, L. O., Gerlach, M. J. M., & Pless, B. S. (1997). *Adult Nursing: Acute and Community Care* (2nd ed.). Stamford, CT: Appleton & Lange.

California Board of Registered Nursing. (1997). *Nursing Practice Act: Rules and Regulations.* Sacramento, CA: State of California Department of Consumer Affairs.

Claiborne, R. (1989). *The Roots of English: A Reader's Handbook of Word Origins.* New York: Anchor.

Fuller, K. (no date). *Documentation.* Torrance, CA: Homestead Schools, Inc.

Hayakawa, S. I. (1964). *Language and Thought* (2nd ed.). New York: Harcourt, Brace & World.

McDonough, J. T., Jr. (Ed.). (1994). *Stedman's Concise Medical Dictionary* (2nd ed.). Baltimore: Williams & Wilkins.

Mosby's Medical, Nursing, and Allied Health Dictionary (4th ed.). (1994). St. Louis: Mosby.

Riverside Webster II Dictionary (Rev. ed.). (1996). New York: Berkeley.

Thomas, C. L. (Ed.). (1997). *Taber's Cyclopedic Medical Dictionary* (18th ed.). Philadelphia: F. A. Davis.

Thompson, J. M., & Wilson, S. F. (1996). *Health Assessment for Nursing Practice.* St. Louis: Mosby.

CHAPTER 1

Introduction

Language is a primary method of communication. Good speaking and writing skills are considered necessary to manage our daily activities. The student works to achieve written and verbal English proficiency in order to progress from one level of education to the next. Grammatically correct and comprehensible language remain constant in education until the student enters nursing school and is immersed in a language within a language. The expectation is that he or she will selectively communicate necessary information to members of the multidisciplinary medical team clearly, objectively, and in an organized, timely manner.

The language used for medical and nursing documentation and for verbal report is remarkably different than most people use in daily conversation. Medical and nursing terms are learned in nursing theory classes. Prioritizing patient data and organizing objective descriptors in a logical sequence is an important skill often learned only through trial and error.

This workbook is designed to assist the novice nurse in building the language skills necessary for clarity in both written and verbal documentation. It is a tool that enables the student nurse to present a professional report to members of the medical team beginning with his or her initial patient contact. By progressing through the exercises, the student learns how to include pertinent information using an organized format, stated in nonbiased language that is specific to a given situation. This workbook could not possibly address every possible situation; however, it does provide guided exercises that the learner can use to develop language skills and practice the professional presentation of patient information.

WHAT'S THE POINT?

The purpose in building language skills for comprehensive documentation is both simple and complex. The obvious reason is to ensure good, effective, and error-free patient care. In fact, the rationale for good documentation includes accurate historical record keeping, medical-legal documentation, information transfer among the health care team, and time-efficient verbal reporting. The use of professional language in an organized format allows the reporter to revisit the written note at any future time and understand the intent and content of the note. Consistent language and format in verbal communication help the reporter to confirm, with reasonable certainty, that the information presented is consistent with the written record.

In a medical care environment, it is necessary to consider reimbursement issues and medical-legal consequences. Exclusions in documentation may indicate observations not made, tasks not performed. The traditional adage is **"not documented, not done."** Without clear and inclusive documentation, it can appear that a patient receiving the best of care may have received none. This does not necessarily indicate an error in nursing practice, but rather in language and methodology used in the documentation process.

EFFICIENT LANGUAGE USE

Throughout the educational process emphasis is placed on the efficient and appropriate use of language to express thoughts, ideas, and observations. You are taught to use rules of English grammar to ensure that you present completed thoughts that can be read and understood. Clerical personnel learn shorthand, a means to record dictation through the use of special symbols, which are then translated back to the original text. Business shorthand is used in order to allow rapid dictation and ensure exact translation. Shorthand notes should be able to be transcribed by anyone who has learned this skill.

The efficient use of language in nursing documentation is likened to using shorthand. The rules of English grammar are often discarded as it is time-consuming and frequently unnecessary to use complete sentences. Nursing shorthand includes all pertinent data necessary to succinctly describe the condition and progress of a patient. Brevity and completeness are the goals. Hence, the need to learn nursing as a second language, focusing upon objective and discreet language.

You, the nursing student, are learning to document data and to prioritize information in a logical order that describes a situation objectively. Your target audiences are future care providers who need comparative data and anyone who may subsequently have need to review the chart. Good documentation should provide clear information that leaves little room for interpretation. Subjective data are limited to direct quotes as necessary.

Learning to use correct descriptive language to present data requires that you develop fluency in a technical vocabulary concurrent with the development of your physical assessment skills. In nursing, you will be confronted with words that have an everyday use as well as specific technical meaning in individual nursing venues. It is often necessary to refer to a medical dictionary, and in some cases a regular dictionary, to check definitions of these commonly used words to ensure proper interpretation.

FORMS, FORMS, FORMS!

Exceptional charting, a policy that assumes all care is complete unless noted, poses a particular challenge to nurses. Institutions attempting to decrease paperwork instate this charting method, supported by task checklists. Nurses, in an effort to accommodate the employer, or in some cases out of frustration related to inadequate space to enter information, may severely restrict written comments. Reliable methodology does exist to ensure inclusion of all the necessary information. Use of such a methodology addresses the objection that narrative notes are inconsistent and therefore unreliable. In fact, consistent use of language in the written note reduces liability that may result from incomplete or vague statements. Specific language and consistent format are the primary tools for this purpose.

FORMAT

Medical schools dominate the format market. Nurses can adapt the reporting style of medical practitioners without losing sight of the nursing focus. The format used by this workbook is in principle the same used in a majority of physical assessment texts. Efforts to work toward consistency in today's health care environment challenge teachers to keep current as reporting styles change. Nurses must adjust to the format used within their work environment and understand that words chosen for documentation and report are important. Remember, there are medical-legal consequences for what is stated, what is not stated, and the language used in documentation. The system for writing and reporting taught in this text is consistent with other contemporary systems.

ADJECTIVES vs. DESCRIPTORS

Adjectives and descriptors modify content. A novelist uses adjectives to enhance storytelling and creatively add to the readers' visualization of the story being told. Nurses use descriptors to objectively describe an event or observation, clarifying current patient status. Descriptors in nursing documentation need to be clearly understood, relate to a specific observation, and be necessary to the record. The descriptors of a symptom describe onset, location, quality, chronology, setting, associated manifestations, alleviating and aggravating factors, and meaning to the patient. The novice nurse frequently rewrites his or her notes in order to eliminate unnecessary, biased, or inaccurate descriptors. This trial and error method is frustrating and time consuming, and may foster an aversion in the nurse to charting.

Written and verbal proficiency take on new meaning for the nursing student. Nurses relate the patient's status without needing a subject, predicate, and object. Prepositions and articles are rarely relevant. There is a definitive need for coherent charting that minimizes the number of words used while clearly stating all details applicable to the patient at the time the note is written.

ABBREVIATIONS

Institutions adopt standardized lists of accepted and routinely used abbreviations. Many are common to institutions around the country. These are used in this workbook's individual case studies. The new nurse retains abbreviations more easily as he or she uses them in context than through rote memorization. Familiarity with commonly accepted abbreviations and those frequently used in individual institutions is essential. The student needs to be aware of variations among schools, hospitals, clinics, and geographical locations.

Some hospitals publish their own lists of commonly used abbreviations. These lists are often several pages long and only become familiar to staff with repetitive use. Checking an institution's manuals for this information is vital, facilitating the nurse's adaptation to new environments without "abbreviation trauma."

GETTING STARTED

Language skills enhance critical thinking skills. This workbook's exercises assist the nurse in isolating and prioritizing information used for reporting and documenting. Like any language, *and nursing is a second language,* practice and repetition reinforce familiarity and fluency. Nursing theory teaches what information is important; this text teaches how to state that information in verbal report and written record. Television actors who portray medical personnel are great at giving a fluid medical verbal report from a script but are challenged to understand what most of the words mean. Nurses know what they need to report and to record, but vacillate over what language to use and how to precisely describe situations. It is the authors' hope that nurses use this text to learn language skills and demystify this action-packed shorthand form of communication.

Remember, this workbook is designed to be a working and useful tool. You may end up with a dog-eared, coffee-stained, ragged text: proof of the nurse's diligence and of the workbook's usefulness!

CHAPTER 2

Nursing as a Second Language

For the purpose of discussion and learning, you will *begin to differentiate* between the common usage of words and their technical application within nursing practice. The workbook refers to words used by laypersons that have meaning in the nonmedical context as *common words*.

Later on, the workbook references common words in terms of their application within the nursing scenario. You are encouraged to check your work as you go along to make sure that you are using common words within the context of their specialized definitions. Your goal is to relate each word to nursing practice rather than to common usage. This is important because the technical, specialized meanings of words are the basis for teaching nursing process and for evaluating a student's comprehension, performance, and competency.

FAMILIAR WORDS

Words in common use among the general public have entirely different meanings when applied to nursing.

Learning these common words and understanding their application within medicine's technical world will help build your conceptual knowledge base.

WORD LIST

accessory	bed	excitement
accommodate	capture	hardware
amplitude	contraction	humor
appendix	conduction	irrigation
appreciate	crown	labor
arrest	discharge	line
articulate	drain	mole
artifact	dress	papoose
bag	eliminate	retention
beat	evacuate	standing

Exercise 2.1

Each item in this chapter's Word List has both a common and technical meaning. Match each word with its corresponding set of definitions and compare the intent or usage of the terms as both common and technical words.

1. _Arrest_
   Common: seize and hold under legal authority
   Technical: stopped, as in organ function or disease process

2. _Mole_
   Common: small mammal; undercover spy
   Technical: small, raised growth on skin; intrauterine mass

3. _Appreciate_
   Common: think well of or value
   Technical: recognize quality of symptom

4. _Contraction_
   Common: shortened word form
   Technical: muscle shortening or an increase in tension; heartbeat; expulsive muscle shortening during labor

5. _Hardware_
   Common: articles made of metal; tools; parts of a computer
   Technical: orthopedic appliances for internal or external use

6. _Eliminate_
   Common: get rid of; to remove
   Technical: expel waste material from body

7. _evacuate_
   Common: withdraw from a hazardous place; vacate
   Technical: empty, especially bowel waste; remove from, as with uterine contents

8. _Articulate_
   Common: well-spoken
   Technical: jointed; surface meeting of joints

9. _Accomodate_
   Common: willing to do a favor; lodging; a convenience
   Technical: state of adjustment or adaptation especially eye focus

10. _Appendix_
    Common: supplemental section at end of book
    Technical: an appendage, most commonly related to the small bowel

11. _Humor_
    Common: ability to be funny, comic
    Technical: fluid or semifluid substance in body

12. _Artifact_
    Common: man-made object, often of historical interest
    Technical: anything caused incidentally by technique used rather than natural occurrence

13. _excitement_
    Common: elicit, provoke
    Technical: potential for stimulation

14. _Accessory_
    Common: something extra but nonessential; someone who helps another break laws
    Technical: auxiliary, as with muscles or nerves

15. _____Bed_____
    Common: sleeping furniture; ground for planting
    Technical: supporting structure for tissue

16. _____beat_____
    Common: hit repeatedly; surpass or defeat
    Technical: stroke or pulsation

17. _____Capture_____
    Common: seize or take possession of by force; represent
    Technical: normal response of heart muscle to electrical impulse

18. _____Crown_____
    Common: ornament; coin; hit or strike on head
    Technical: top or highest part of organ; presentation of baby's head in birth canal; dental prosthesis

19. _____Dress_____
    Common: to put on clothes; one-piece style of woman's apparel
    Technical: apply cover to support or protect wound

20. _____drain_____
    Common: draw off liquid; channel or pipe; to empty
    Technical: tube to remove discharge or fluid from cavity

21. _____Retention_____
    Common: hold, keep possession of; to hire
    Technical: keeping body waste normally, as with urine

22. _____Bag_____
    Common: flexible container; to grab or capture; area of interest
    Technical: pouch or container to hold and/or measure body fluids or drainage

23. _____Papoose_____
    Common: Native American infant
    Technical: method for restraining a child for a procedure

24. _____Line_____
    Common: narrow continuous mark; boundary; covering for an interior surface
    Technical: access cannula for vascular testing or medicating

25. _____Standing_____
    Common: positioned upright
    Technical: prepared instructions to be performed automatically under specific conditions

26. _____Amplitude_____
    Common: great size; fullness
    Technical: measure of an action potential

27. _____Conduction_____
    Common: to lead; to transmit
    Technical: transmission of energy from one point to another

28. _____Discharge_____
    Common: relieve of a burden or task; to fire from a job
    Technical: secretion or excretion of a body fluid; release from care

29. _____Labor_____
    Common: work or task; those who do work for others for wages
    Technical: effort expended for activity as breathing; process of delivering fetus

30. _____Irrigate_____
    Common: to water, artificially
    Technical: to wash wound with saline or medicated fluids

COMMON TERMS/UNFAMILIAR DEFINITIONS

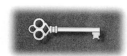

Upon hearing common language used in the context of patient care, you may initially experience some confusion. In fact, some of these words and phrases may seem like puns.

For example, imagine how the phrases in Exercise 2.2 might be misinterpreted by someone who is not familiar with the specific language use.

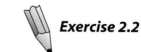

Exercise 2.2

Match the phrases with their meaning in the health care setting. For example, the answer to (1) "Piggyback the antibiotic" is G.

1. "Piggyback the antibiotic" G
2. "Empty the bag"   - E
3. "Answer the radio"   - O
4. "Papoose the patient"   - H
5. "Start a line"   - R
6. "Measure the response" I
7. "Write standing orders" B
8. "Take down the order" L
9. "Push it"- A
10. "The appy in room 4" - C
11. "Do the treatment before the meal" S
12. "Decrease procedure turnover time" P
13. "Determine acuity"   - J
14. "Check the crash cart"- K
15. "Answer the call light" Q
16. "Dangle the patient" - D
17. "Flush the line"   —   M
18. "Prepare a cutdown tray" F
19. "Send it to the M & M committee" - N

A. Deliver medication IV push according to the order or acceptable method of delivery

B. Write standard orders proscribing action for a specified situation

C. Refer to patient by diagnosis (appendectomy) or current complaint and room number; not an appropriate way to describe individual patients

D. Help the patient to sit at side of bed with legs dangling, often for a specific amount of time, while assessing the patient's ability to tolerate this intervention; not the same as "up in chair"

E. Empty and measure contents of receptacle, such as catheter bag, colostomy bag, or drain

F. Prepare for a procedure to start an IV by exposing the vein surgically, usually when a patient's veins are extremely difficult to access through the usual IV procedure

G. Deliver a medication by superimposing a secondary IV set up on the existing line

H. Restrain patient, usually an infant or toddler, in a papoose-style protective restraint

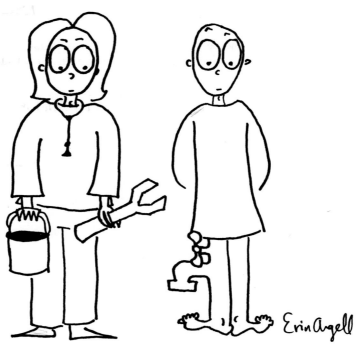

Checking the Drain

I. Assess and quantify the patient's response to medication or treatment

J. Review the number of nursing hours spent performing necessary care in order to assign patients to units or teams and to assess staffing needs

K. Inventory the cart containing supplies for emergency use; stock missing supplies and replace outdated meds and instruments

L. Transcribe a verbal order into the patient's chart

M. Deliver a medicated or plain clearing agent to a patient's IV line to ensure that it is, or remains, patent and effective

N. Refer incident or outcome to the Morbidity and Mortality Committee for review

O. Respond to radio contact with health providers in the field

P. Decrease the amount of costly time spent between procedures cleaning and setting up for subsequent room use

Q. Respond to the patient's call signal or emergency light in a room, usually within a specified time frame, which may be determined by law

R. Initiate IV access for fluid replacement or medication delivery

S. Plan an intervention prior to the patient's next meal

Some of the phrases sound "funny," some seem disrespectful of a serious situation, and others simply appear to be nonsense.

LEARNING THE LANGUAGE

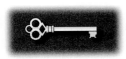

In theoretical and clinical instruction, it is often presumed that you, the student, have prior knowledge and command of nursing's technical language. The core content of a general nursing curriculum does not necessarily provide teaching hours to explain the language of nursing. Time is more likely to be spent teaching application of the technical language to the nursing process.

Language is the core of spoken and written communications. Its proper use is emphasized throughout the educational process. Once you enter nursing school, word usage and grammatical clarifications are generally provided to you by your instructor in retrospect, commonly by reviewing your nursing documentation efforts, in a manner that "corrects" your improper word selection or application. At this important juncture a change may be effected only if you, as a student, understand the "corrected" word selection's more technical application. If your root comprehension of the incorrect word or of its technical application is lacking, you may simply adjust the error at the time, but repeat the mistake later on. The adaptation of common language and the subsequent incorporation of the technical application is not automatic.

The correlation between correction and adaptation happens frequently in the clinical setting in the review of your nursing documentation efforts. It is an opportune "teaching moment," and as nursing instruction progresses, you are potentially on a circular path of error. An improper selection or application is made, the instructor provides you a technical word usage option, the correction is made, another retrospective correction is offered after an improper selection is made, and the loop continues.

You perhaps end up in a situation of never having *identified* the basis of your technical language use deficit while at the same time being expected to participate in nursing education's dynamic learning process. This learning process is built consecutively upon a foundation of technical knowledge as well as its proper application in the clinical setting.

Time limits the instruction periods to prioritizing the theoretical content necessary to the nursing process, leaving the practical application entirely to lab and clinical settings. Details of charting style and language use may only be addressed minimally and for a specific circumstance, as time permits.

Interactions between you and your instructor often occur in your clinical section. By nature they are "in the moment," and may not readily identify fundamental deficits in language usage or technical application. This is not to say that the learning system is flawed, but that this particular teaching style requires that your comprehension and preparation for technical language use must be in place. The clinical nature of the corrective process does not ensure substantive changes in your comprehension.

 Exercise 2.3

Read the following charting selection and review the words in the phrase for technical meaning.

 Example:

"assess ADLs for discharge planning"

Assess: the caregiver observed and evaluated the patient's ability to perform basic daily tasks for himself or herself

ADL: acronym for activities of daily living: self care and hygiene, mobility, basic understanding of posthospitalization activity recommendation

Discharge planning: Prior to the patient's going home or being discharged from the facility, typically a plan of action is developed to determine if a patient needs something to ensure a safe recovery at home

Following the example above, isolate words and phrases that require specific and technical language skills for correct application. A detailed explanation of each phrase is included in italics.

1. "Transpose new bag of solution into existing line and run @ 100 an hour" *(The nurse will take down the former IV solution bag and replace it with a new bag of IV solution to be infused at the rate of 100 cc per hour.)*

   Transpose - take down former IV bag And Replace w/ New IV @ 100 an Hour - infused @ rate of 100 c. per hr.

2. "Measure the pt's I & O and force fluids if output less than 50 cc per hr" *(The caregiver is requested to monitor and measure the patient's oral and parenteral intake and urinary output. If the patient voids less than 50 cc per hour the caregiver is ordered to increase the patient's fluid intake.)*

   pts. = patient I & O = Intake & Output
   measure I/O (IV/Oral Input - Urinary Output)
   If pts voids > 50cc ↑ pts. fluids intake.

3. "Titrate to maintain the BP @ 90 systolic" *(The nurse is to regulate the flow of IV fluids or IV medication drip to keep the patient's systolic blood pressure measurement at no less than 90 mm Hg.)*

   Titrate - regulate flow of IV Fluids/Meds
   BP = Blood pressure
   @ 90 - maintain BP No less than 90

4. "Turn, cough and deep breathe the pt. q 2h" *(The caregiver is to assist the patient to turn side to side every two hours. While turning the patient side to side the caregiver is also to instruct the patient to take three deep breaths inward and to expel the last deep breath in the form of a cough.)*

   Turn - turn side to side @ 2H
   Cough/Deep breath - 3 deep breath, last breath Cough
   Q2H = Every two Hours

5. "Adjust O2 from 1 L, to room air 15 min q hr" *(The nurse is to adjust the O2 delivery system to room air for 15 minutes out of each hour, or on an hourly basis. The nurse will assess the patient's adaptation to this routine.)*

   O2 = Oxygen   q Hr = Every Hour.
   1L - One liter of O2
   - 15 minutes of RA every Hour - on Hourly Basis.

6. "Keep patient NPO and supine following the spinal study" *(The caregiver is to withhold oral fluids and to keep the patient flat on his or her back in bed after a test in which the patient's spinal column is accessed.)*

   NPO - Nothing by mouth
   Supine - flat on back
   Spinal study - test in which spinal column is Assessed

TECHNICAL DEFINITIONS

Technical terms are words specific to professional use; they may also have non-technical meanings. Contextual understanding of such words is vital, and interpretation may be needed.

Medical and legal concerns require that nursing place an emphasis on language specific to its professional use. Differentiation in a word's meaning and discrimination as to its proper usage are incumbent to your safe and legal standard of practice. In language's common use, often vague statements are intentionally used to convey or imply a meaning subject to the reader's interpretation. In nursing documentation, vague language subject to interpretation is a dangerous practice.

In verbal communication the emphasis on any single word in a given statement is used to inject accurate, exaggerated, or artificial meaning into the message. However documentation is a written form of communication. It is without the benefit or bias of your voice inflection. Emphasis, therefore, must be attained through cuttingly objective and accurate descriptors in the written narrative.

This adds additional responsibility for you to objectively and thoroughly note circumstances and assessments regarding an individual patient's care. Written notes do not permit you the opportunity to emphasize those words in a statement that can assist in the accurate portrayal of events. Charting must reflect, all in transcribed silence, the circumstances in an objective, professional, and impartial manner.

Tone, volume, and cadence are three tools commonly associated with verbal communication. The goal of clear, concise, written communication is to use words that accomplish these tasks in a silent medium. Relating the exact words of a patient is always permitted. These words must be direct quotes within quotation marks. It is not appropriate to enclose an *interpretation* of the patient's remark in quotation marks.

Exercise 2.4

This exercise demonstrates how verbal emphasis on an individual word may alter the meaning of the whole phrase. Read each phrase several times, placing the emphasis on different key words with each reading. For fun, exaggerate the emphasis on each word. Listen to how each statement can be altered simply by inflection and emphasis. Imagine this process applied to the nursing notes you write!

Example:

Say, "I didn't say the test was stupid," with no emphasis, or flat intonation.
Now, emphasize the boldface word.

"**I** didn't say the test was stupid."
"I **didn't** say the test was stupid."
"I didn't **say** the test was stupid."
"I didn't say the **test** was stupid."
"I didn't say the test was **stupid**."

Repeat the exercise with the following phrases. You can also make up your own phrases or think of instances when you have used inflection and emphasis to make a point in everyday conversation.

1. "He didn't hear what I said."
2. "You can't try that with me."
3. "Will you stop and listen to me?"
4. "Everything he did seemed to make things better."
5. "You never listen to what I say."

In nursing, there is almost no indication for vague assertions other than those in quotation marks that have been related directly by the patient and are relative to the patient's care. This is not to say that it will be easy for you to eliminate imprecise statements in the patient's legal record of care.

Consider these questions:

Is the subjectivity and imprecise documentation a habit of the individual?

Is it a prior common language practice?

Is it reflective of a fundamental lack of comprehension and contextual adaptation to the technical world of the nursing language?

It is likely that all nurses have at one time or another entered subjective and nonspecific statements into the patient's record. As nursing practice has evolved from physician's bedside helpmate to an independent professional as well as technical and deductive practice, so too has the requirement for more precise and objective notations in the patient's record of care. The emphasis is to quantify rather than qualify observations, to record accurately a sequence of events surrounding the patient's care, and to do so in a manner that would reflect, even years later the definitive and clinical nature of the patient's status and the nature and outcome of care received.

Nurse educators have recognized this vital precept and know what textbooks to require, what words to teach. If the presumption of learning foregoes your basic language preparation for the use of technical terms, you may or may not learn how to discriminate or decide what terms are acceptable and truly applicable in a given situation. Similarly, an experienced nurse, not yet adapted to the current demands in documentation, may not know to differentiate between subjective and selective, between quantify and qualify, in terms of words with common language patterns.

 Exercise 2.5

Consider and review the following nonspecific, or vague, samples frequently seen in narrative entries in nursing records. Evaluate them based on their intent, but review them for their legal validity and professional discrimination.

1. "pt. slept through noc"

   _____

   _____

   _____

2. "complains of slight pain with palpation"

   _____

   _____

   _____

3. "tolerated procedure well"

   _____

   _____

   _____

4. "appears in no distress"

   _____

   _____

   _____

5. "resting comfortably when checked hourly"

_____

_____

_____

MEMORIZATION AND THE LEARNING PROCESS

In learning the definition of a medical term not commonly used in everyday language, you may at first use a process of memorization. This would be followed by gradual assimilation, comprehension, and application. If you lack the basic ability to assimilate within the learning process then the term is simply memorized, and adequate comprehension of its application and adaptation may not occur.

This may reflect an overall weakness in the learning structure as you attempt to differentiate between common or technical meanings. When brought together with the brisk-paced and dynamic nature of nursing's didactic core content, it is easy to understand why some students may excel and others struggle. Most of us can memorize tables for addition and subtraction. If we do not understand what addition and subtraction symbols themselves mean, then we are relegated to remain within the memorization realm.

 Exercise 2.6

Check both your retention of the words presented at the beginning of this chapter and your application skills. Match a word from the word list with the correct medical definition.

stopcock   local
dilate   cardiac catheter
IV catheter   junction
joint   catheter
radiation   dress
anterior   fundus
stream   urinary catheter
obtunded

1. a tube passed through an opening in the body or through the skin to take fluids out of the body or to put fluids into a body area _Catheter_

2. small plastic tube inserted through the skin into an artery or vein to insert fluids or medications or to measure circulatory pressures _IV Catheter_

3. long plastic tube inserted through the skin into a vein large enough to permit passage of the tube directly into the heart chambers. Used in a cardiac catheterization to provide visualization of the workings inside of the heart _Cardiac Catherization_

4. a short rubber or latex tube passed through the urethral opening in order to empty urine from the bladder or to instill fluids into the bladder and make it full _Urinary Catheter_

5. an anatomical term used to describe location, in this case, top, front, or in front of _Anterior_

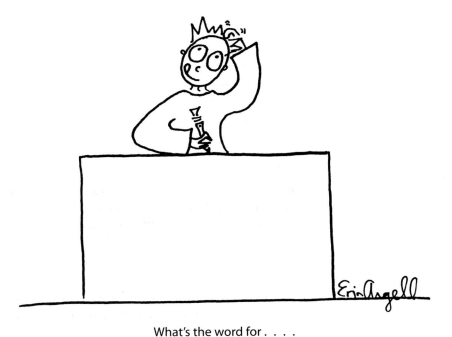

What's the word for . . . .

6. to broaden, stretch, expand, open. May be used with an organ, cavity, or opening in the body ___dilate___

7. the term for a place where two bones touch and whose end points are joined ___Joint___

8. place where two parts or two tissues or two layers of body substance come together ___Junction___

9. a small, valve-like, plastic adapter that is added to permit control of the flow of fluids, to monitor pressures within circulation, or to permit access to more than one fluid line into a catheter _____

10. the largest portion of a hollow organ, which also is the furthest point from the organ's opening ___Fundus___

11. a loss of responsiveness, alertness, or sensation. May refer to state of consciousness or state of progressing and severe respiratory distress _____

12. something used to close over, to provide shielding, or to wrap a wound or opening on the body's surface ___Dress___

13. limited to one area; used as liquid medication to affect sensation in a specific part; designates a specific site where infection has or may occur ___local___

14. a flow of liquid from or into the body ___Stream___

15. a general term for an emanation or divergence of energy, heat, beam, element, or fluorescent light ___Radiation___

Stopcock
Obtunded

NURSING APPLICATION

You will be better prepared to apply the nursing process if preliminary specialized language skills are mastered concurrent with or prior to your mastery of the theoretical nursing content. As related earlier, language must be specific to its technical use. You are required to assimilate as part of the learning process an ability to both differentiate and discriminate among the choices of technical terms available. At the brisk pace that didactic content is presented to you, there is little time to review language skills, particularly those dedicated to documentation, while discussing theoretical content.

Exercise 2.7

The following phrases might be introduced in either a didactic or clinical setting. They require an understanding of the exact words used and the ability to interpret the intent of the words and their application in a clinical setting. Read the following phrases and try to paraphrase the noted action. Compare your answer with the actual meaning of the phrase.

1. "the nurse turned up the amplitude in order to better visualize the waveforms"

   _____
   _____
   _____

2. "the pt was instructed on discharge teaching to carefully empty his bladder"

   _____
   _____
   _____

3. "the consent called for open fixation with internal reduction"

   _____
   _____
   _____

4. "a pt. elopement could bring up questions about pt. abandonment"

   _____
   _____
   _____

5. "the integrity of the globe was unaffected and the humor remained intact"

   _____
   _____
   _____

6. "healing had progressed to where the pt. had laid down a new capillary bed"

   _____
   _____
   _____

7. "failure to capture the beat concerned the MD"

   _____
   _____
   _____

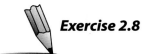

Exercise 2.8

This exercise contains incomplete action, or application, phrases common to the clinical setting. Check your understanding of how some of the words introduced in this chapter and common in everyday practice are applied.

Make a selection from the word list to complete the following phrase.

accommodation	conduction
exquisite	catheter
atrophy	standing orders
radiated	pattern
arrest	eliminate
reduction	crown
accessory	papoose
fundus	

[handwritten margin notes: Exquisite, standing orders, fundus]

1. A code was called due to cardiac ___Arrest___
2. Anesthesia was necessary for the _____ of the fracture
3. Palpation of abdomen resulted in ___Reduction___ tenderness
4. Noted labored respiration with use of ___Accesory___ muscles
5. The pupils reacted to light and ___Accomodation___
6. Pain ___radiated___ to the left arm and jaw
7. The EKG measures ___Conduction___ of impulses
8. The _____ was 10 cm
9. Muscle showed marked ___Atrophy___
10. The nurse explained the procedure prior to inserting a ___Catheter___
11. Measurement of the ___Crown___ of the baby's head showed normal growth
12. The patient was instructed to use the bathroom to ___eliminate___ and obtain a specimen
13. She found a set of _____ in the patient's admission packet.
14. The technician assisted the MD to secure the infant with a ___papoose___ for the procedure.
15. There was a ___pattern___ of irregularity demonstrated by the EKG.

SPELLING

Correct spelling in charting is absolutely necessary to ensure that subsequent readers understand and interpret documented notes correctly. Words commonly used in charting can often sound alike but have entirely unrelated meanings. This holds true for pronunciation during verbal report. Names and words may have more than one accepted pronunciation. It is important to be true to the pronunciation accepted and understood in your current clinical setting. Variations in meaning may affect care and can negatively affect a patient's recovery.

Spelling and pronunciation can alter the interpretation of an assessment. Potential medication errors are always a risk if the transcriber is a careless speller or does not double check a verbal or written order or if there is any confusion with the pronunciation or spelling of a word. Experienced nurses double check orders

---

BOX 2.1

Suffixes and Prefixes

In English classes you may have learned about the root origin of words and about the use of suffixes and prefixes. Continue your learning! How a word originates can be very helpful in building a vocabulary in medical terminology. Technical meanings can mislead you if you are not sure of the correct word root.

A way to learn about root words is to browse through your medical dictionary or glossary in your text. Locate a section where words have similar prefixes, such as "hemi-," "hem-" or "hema-". The prefix "hemi-" means one-half or partial, while "hem-" and "hema-" mean blood. Consider the magnitude of error that misinterpreting a single word could cause. If you aren't sure what a word means or if you aren't sure about the root always look it up.

Suffixes may also be helpful to determine the meaning of a word. The suffixes "-itis" and "-osis" often follow common root words. Look up the words "diverticulitis" and "diverticulosis." The word root is "diverticula." The suffix "-itis" means inflammation of a diverticula, while the suffix "-osis" indicates presence of or increase in the number of diverticula.

Practice with daily language use helps you to determine what a word means. By dissecting and analyzing unfamiliar words to determine their meaning, you continue to gain proficiency in language. You may also benefit by reviewing unfamiliar words in a dictionary or text. It can be helpful to look in a dictionary of common words to see what words with the same root, prefix, or suffix are included.

It is customary to have both medical and common dictionaries available for staff reference. Become familiar with the features of the available dictionary. This tool supports good nursing process and accurate documentation practice.

that they suspect may be incorrect based upon their knowledge of the patient's diagnosis and symptoms.

Note the following words which are similar in pronunciation and/or spelling but which have unrelated meanings:

abdominal/abominable

Zantac/Xanax

content/contempt

bacteriostatic/ bactericidal

hemoglobin/ hemoglobinemia

hemostasis/homeostasis

incisor/incisure

keratin/carotene

cervix/cervical

epinephrine/ephedrine

glucagon/glycogen

perineum/peritoneum

HANDWRITING

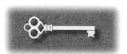

The best note can be misleading if the reader has to guess what as written and cannot clearly interpret the note. While many comments are jokingly made about physician's handwriting and the difficulty in reading their orders, this is not a laughing matter. Poor handwriting can, at the least, delay patient care while you verify the intent of the order. Medication errors are often related to undecipherable handwriting.

Coordinating patient care leading to maximum wellness is a goal that challenges the health care team under the best of circumstances. This is best accomplished when easily avoidable errors related to spelling and handwriting are eliminated from the care equation (Figs. 2.1 to 2.4).

Figure 2.1

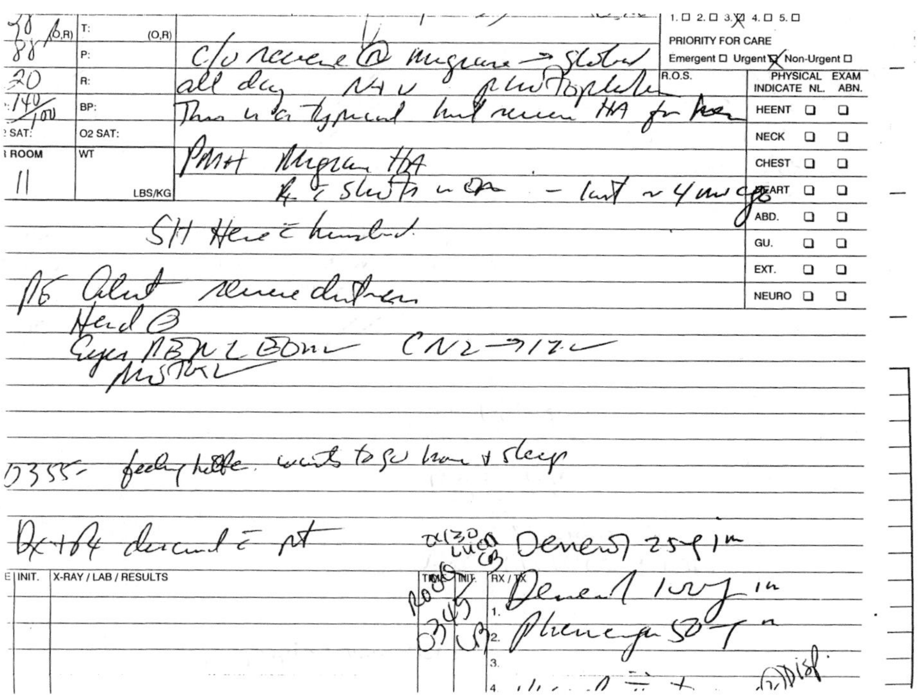

Challenging handwriting sample.

Figure 2.2

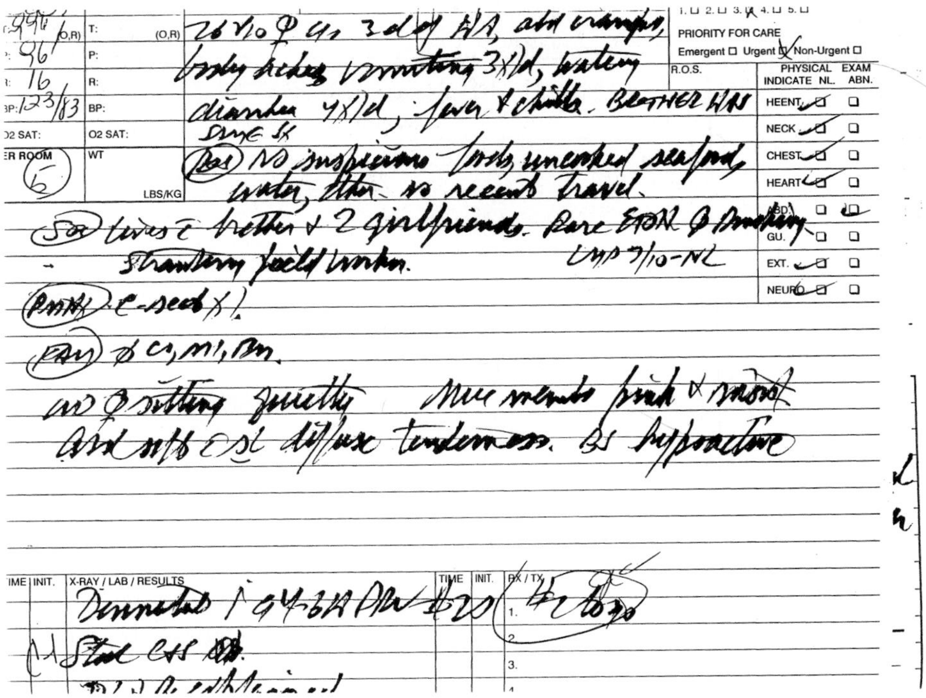

Challenging handwriting sample.

Figure 2.3

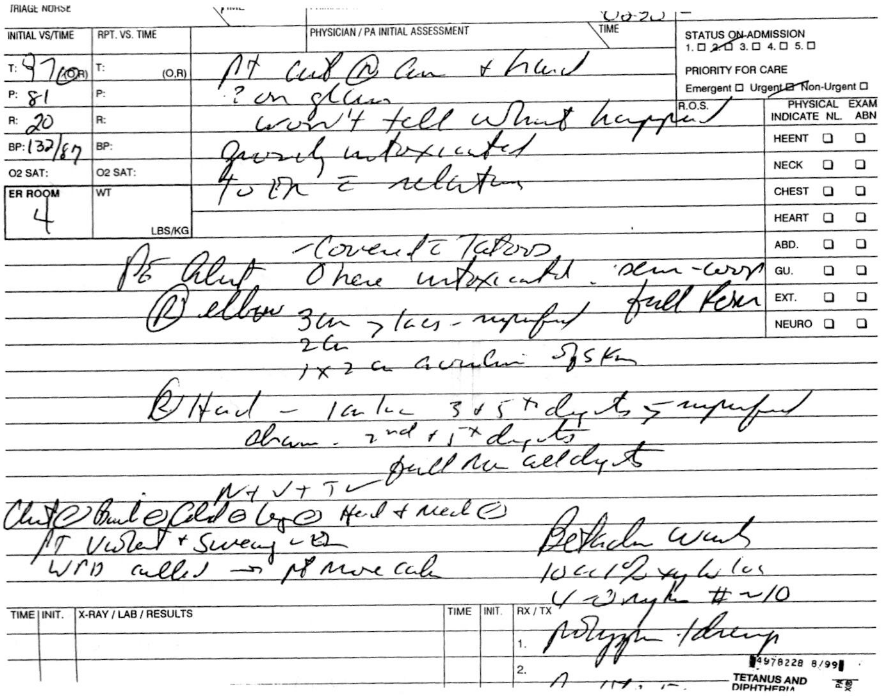

Challenging handwriting sample.

Figure 2.4

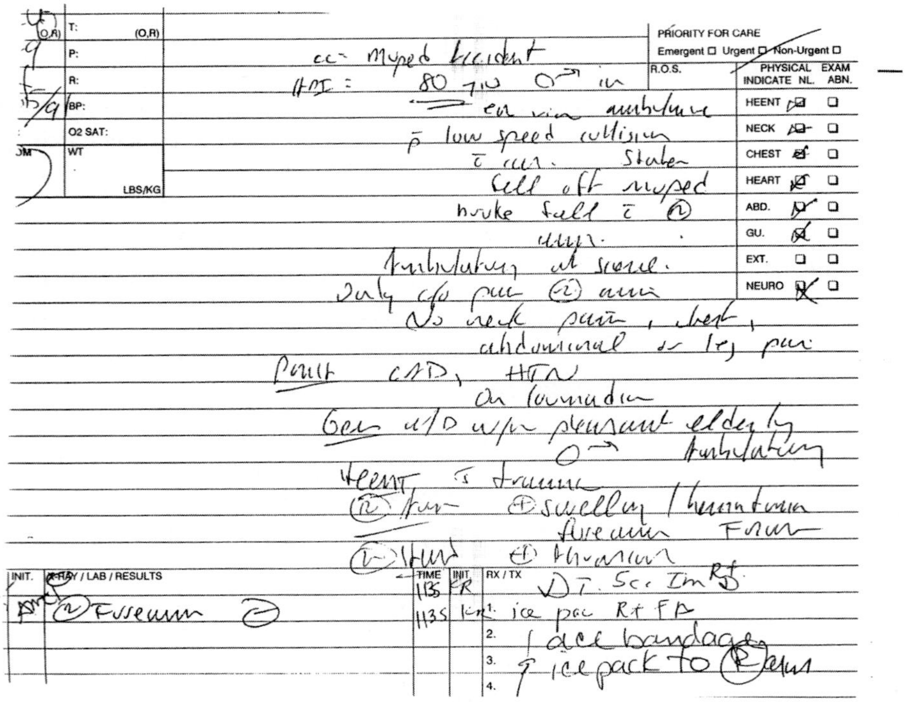

Challenging handwriting sample.

The medical legal implications related to spelling errors will be addressed in more detail Chapter 8.

PATIENT CARE IMPACT

It is clear that understanding language, its technical use and meaning, and pronouncing and spelling words correctly directly affects patient care. Descriptive words chosen to represent patient status and current needs should be objective and specific. The patient is not expected to know the medical terms appropriate to their experience. It is a nursing responsibility to investigate a comment or complaint in order to determine what is going on with a patient *right now*. A patient's subjective complaint is often best recorded as a direct quote. The nurse follows up by investigating the complaint and soliciting descriptive and quantifying details from the patient.

For example, a patient may state he is feeling "uncomfortable." You, the nurse who is evaluating the stated discomfort, must explore what that means, isolate the origin of the discomfort, and quantify the effect on the patient using a measurable and consistent scale. A chart entry reading "1030: patient feels uncomfortable" says nothing useful for assessment or treatment. Care cannot be planned, implemented, or evaluated based on this scant data. Compare this to the following note. "1030: complains of pain left hip, 4/10 on 1–10 scale, sitting." or written "c/o pain L hip, 4/10 (1–10), sitting." This gives any reader a clearer picture of what, when, and how much.

Commonly used scales to quantify a subjective symptom, and descriptors that quantify, such as "mild, moderate, severe, and exquisite" bring into focus a fuzzy picture because they are universally used and represent a range of intensity commonly understood by health care providers. This demonstrates how even subjective symptoms have objective parameters that can be written in documentary shorthand that is easily interpreted by most providers.

 Exercise 2.9

Evaluate the following comments and determine what missing information would help you to assess the patient's immediate complaint. Choose general areas of information such as "exact location" and "how much"; you will do detailed exercises on descriptors later in the workbook.

1. "My stomach hurts"

   _____

   _____

   _____

2. "I have a headache"

   _____

   _____

   _____

3. "I can't get up"

   _____

   _____

   _____

4. "I feel dizzy"

   _____

   _____

   _____

5. "My feet feel funny"

_____

_____

_____

SHORTHAND, ABBREVIATIONS, PICTURES

Individual health care facilities publish lists of accepted abbreviations for use by the staff. In your nursing practice, it is necessary for you to use them appropriately. These will vary from setting to setting and it is important to conform to your current practice area.

Symbols which have common meanings are used to save valuable time and space. Vague symbols are inappropriate. For instance, a wavy line over an equal sign ≅ traditionally indicates an approximation, expressed as "around," "about," or "sort of." Objective data cannot be documented in this inexact manner. A blood pressure "around" 150/90 connotes an inexact value and is an extremely poor record of patient data.

Here are some of the symbols common to nursing practice and written documentation. Do you know which ones are used by more than one profession? Which are primarily used in health care settings? Practice using the symbols in the space created in your workbook.

CHANGE

The triangle shape represents the word "change" or means "changed to." In mathematics the triangle shape appears as three dots ∴ to note a "change computation." In written notes a lined-in triangle Δ (Fig. 2.5) represents the word "change." Using this symbol saves space and time.

Figure 2.5

CHANGE

ARROWS

Arrows indicating a specific direction can be substituted for words or groups of words. An arrow pointed upward ↑ (Fig. 2.6) indicates an increase in a parameter such as blood pressure, or an amount of drainage. Therefore, "increased blood pressure" can be written ↑BP.

Figure 2.6

INCREASED

A downward arrow ↓ (Fig. 2.7) indicates a decrease or trend in a lower direction, as in ↓ systolic blood pressure.

BOX 2.2

Some Common Abbreviations

Using common word substitutions in charting makes your note easier to read and understand. You should by now be comfortable with using all of the following in your documentation. Capitalization may change the interpretation. For example "os" is the word for an opening as in the cervical os, OS stands for left eye. "OD" is more complicated meaning "right eye," "overdose," or "doctor of optometry" (and not to be confused with "DO," or "osteopath") so context is important.

d	day
qd	every day
bid	twice a day
qid	four times per day
qh	each hour
prn	as needed
po	by mouth, or oral
$\bar{p}$	after
a	before
OS	left eye
OD	right eye
hx	history
dx	diagnosis
re:	regarding, about
$\bar{c}$	with
$\bar{s}$	without
q	each, every

Figure 2.7

DECREASED

The horizontal arrow → (Fig. 2.8) is often used to represent the words "leads to" or "leading to." Concepts in physiology can be "mapped" or demonstrated using words separated by horizontal arrows. The direction of the arrow depicts the progress of an intervention or the expected progression of the disease process. While not usually seen in documentation notes, learning the technique of using horizontal arrows is helpful in deductive thinking and mastering pathophysiology.

Figure 2.8

LEADS TO

POSITIVE AND NEGATIVE

The plus sign alone + or within a circle (Fig. 2.9) symbolizes the word *positive*. In a systems review a plus sign preceding a symptom or condition indicates that either the patient states, or the patient's history shows that the "positive" data are, or have in the past been, positively identified.

Figure 2.9

POSITIVE

The minus sign alone − or within a circle (Fig. 2.10) symbolizes the word *negative*. This symbol indicates that the patient states, or records indicate, no known or current history of this factor or symptom.

Figure 2.10

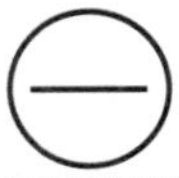

NEGATIVE

The positive and negative symbols are used to identify data derived from lab work or other quantifying sources. The nurse uses the data when determining the patient's needs or assessing the progress of care. Physicians or nurses use the data to reach a diagnosis for the patient. Pertinent or relevant negatives are often included when documenting patient progress in your nursing notes. They help to determine cause of condition or progress of intervention. "No fever" is an example of relevant "pertinent negative" included in a note.

FIGURES

Stick figures can be used to indicate the positioning of a patient during an assessment, interview, or procedure. You may use them when documenting blood pressures, especially if the patient's blood pressure varies with position (e.g., orthostatic changes).

Figures 2.11, 2.12, and 2.13 are the figures most frequently associated with patient positioning.

Figure 2.11

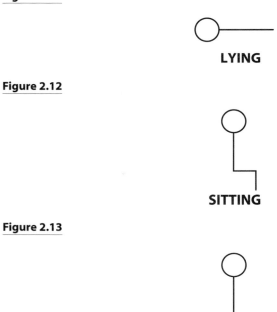

LYING

Figure 2.12

SITTING

Figure 2.13

STANDING

Using stick figures to represent patient position saves you time. It allows you to fully document a procedure even if the documentation space is limited.

REFLEXES

Stick figures are used in documenting reflex checks. A small picture can be used to record the reflex points you have assessed and whether the reflexes appeared

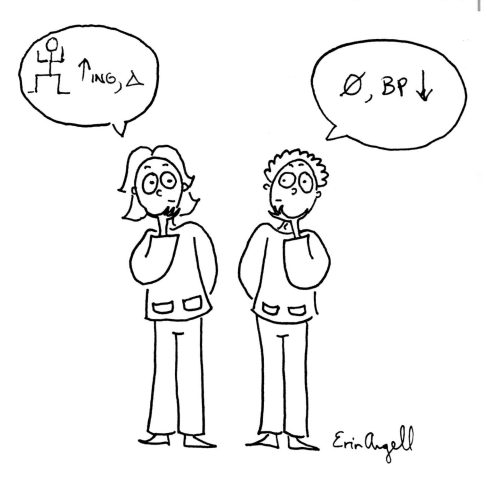

normal, hyper-, or hyporeflexive. For example, +2 is most often considered "normal" when using the numeric scale of 1–4 (Fig. 2.14).

Figure 2.14

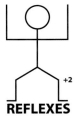

REFLEXES

NO/NOT

Using zero with a slash mark through it ∅ (Fig. 2.15) is commonly used instead of writing "no" or "not." The zero and the minus symbols are not precisely the same and are not necessarily interchangeable. The use of the zero or minus symbols requires discrimination by the practitioner.

Figure 2.15

NO / NOT

BOX 2.3

Avoiding Error

Approved abbreviations are used in many clinical areas. Many abbreviations are common to facilities across the country. It is necessary for practitioners to become fluent in the use of abbreviations, as they are effective aids in time management and efficient use of documentation space. Abbreviations or interpretations may vary depending upon the setting. Be aware of the meaning and use in your current practice setting.

Tx and *Rx* are abbreviations that may create confusion if interpreted incorrectly. For example, in an orthopedic unit *tx* is frequently used in place of the word *traction*; in a walk-in clinic, *tx* might be used in place of the word *treatment*. Similarly, *Rx* is com-

monly expected to mean *prescription*; in a SOAP note, however, it may replace *P* to denote *plan*.

To ensure that care providers reading your written notes are not confused by what you have documented, review your facilities list of accepted abbreviations and comply with written policy.

You are responsible for the clarity of your charting. A note that reads "tx = bedrest $\times$ 3 days" is confusing. If the facility recognizes *tx* to signify *traction*, the note makes no sense at all.

Abbreviations are an appropriate and helpful tool. Always use them in compliance with accepted practice specific to your clinical area and care facility.

LAB VALUES

Medical providers use the following diagrams to record frequently evaluated lab values. The following diagrams are commonly used by providers and are an excellent shorthand tool for nurses. Practice using the diagrams (Figs. 2.16, 2.17, 2.18) by writing in appropriate lab values in the correct space. This is a good time to practice using normal values.

Figure 2.16

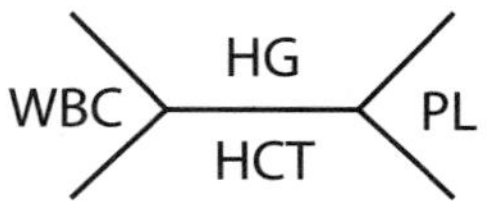

Figure 2.17

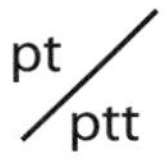

Figure 2.18

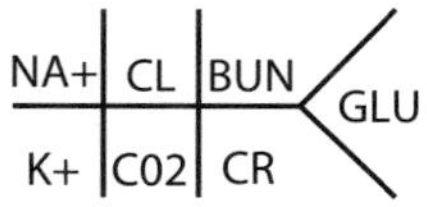

An experienced nurse not familiar with this technique may deduce from the represented numbers which lab tests are noted. To know with certainty which values are recorded can only result from actually learning the technique. You, a student, may not have not had enough exposure to have the easy familiarity with lab values that allows you to associate certain numeric values with specific lab tests.

QUADRANTS

The most common use of the quadrant symbol is in describing the abdomen. The following two examples (Figs. 2.19, 2.20) are commonly accepted ways to anatomically divide and describe the abdomen.

Figure 2.19

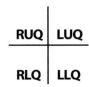

Figure 2.20

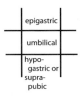

Quadrant description is pertinent and helpful when documenting bowel sounds, abdominal pain, subcutaneous injection sites, or location of fetal heart tones.

GREATER THAN/LESS THAN

Mathematical symbols are used here in place of words. It is one of the more confusing symbols for people to remember. Confusion is most often due to a lack of familiarity and infrequent use.

"Greater than" is an arrowhead symbol that points to the right or toward a parameter > (Fig. 2.21). "Less than" is an arrowhead symbol that points to the left or away from a parameter < (Fig. 2.22). These symbols are frequently used when entering the parameters for numeric lab values or blood pressures. These parameters are often associated with treatment modalities known as "sliding scale regimens," i.e., "hold vasopressor if BP

Figure 2.21

Greater Than

Figure 2.22

Less Than

< 140/80." Blood pressure levels, blood sugars, anticoagulant and seizure medication blood levels often are associated with such sliding scale medication schedules.

Exercise 2.10

This simple exercise is designed to help you recognize greater or lesser comparisons. You must associate each comparison with its correct and corresponding arrowhead symbol. It is important to determine if the arrowhead is pointing toward or away from a value or parameter.

Remember, a symbol with the arrowhead pointing toward a parameter indicates *greater than* (>). An arrowhead pointing away from a value indicates *less than* (<). Complete the following sentences by entering the arrowhead pointing in the correct direction.

1. The size of a mountain is _____>_____ a molehill.
2. A private's rank is _____<_____ a general's rank.
3. The salary of a chief executive is _____>_____ the salary of an assembly line worker.
4. The number 1,000,000 is _____>_____ the number .0000001.
5. A preschooler's weight is _____<_____ the weight of her father.
6. She was exhausted by the 26th mile of the marathon. The effort was much _____>_____ she anticipated.
7. A creek's water volume is _____<_____ the volume of an ocean.
8. The size of a rhinoceros is _____>_____ the size of a koala bear.
9. The height of a tree is _____<_____ the height of the Empire State Building.

The "greater than" and "less than" symbols with a line beneath the arrowhead are used to include "or equal to" for a specified parameter. The symbol for "greater than or equal to" looks like ≥ (Fig. 2.23); "less than or equal to" appears as ≤ (Fig. 2.24). This is an instance in which recording a parameter incorrectly may greatly affect appropriate care.

Figure 2.23

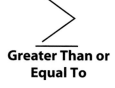

Greater Than or Equal To

Figure 2.24

Less Than or Equal To

DEGREES OF MOTION

Figure 2.25 represents degrees of motion or position. The symbols are not commonly used unless a very detailed record is necessary. Even so, you should have a working knowledge of them.

Figure 2.25

Pictures can be drawn to document the size or location of an observation. Pictures can be worth a thousand words while taking up little charting space. Your art need not be very creative. A picture documenting location and measurements of an infected incision site (Fig. 2.26) can be used to document the progress of wound healing.

Figure 2.26

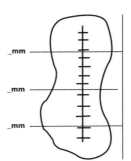

incision site redness with
area affected and measured
for future comparison

Using symbols or glyphs for documentation is not productive if your facility chooses not to recognize them. The triangle used in place of the word *change* or arrows as increase and decrease are commonly used and understood.

Use symbols and glyphs to conserve space and time. It is unnecessary to use prepositions and articles with them. Phrases like "nurse observed" or "patient states" are usually not necessary with each entry. Chapter 8 goes into more detail about vague chart entries.

WHAT YOU SHOULD INCLUDE

An initial interview with a patient includes a health history and all pertinent information regarding the current admission or complaint. If you are a beginning student, you may not have the interviewing skills or the medical knowledge to fully conduct this interview.

What should you include in your note if your skills are limited to hearing and recording patient statements? Include the patient's complaint, your action, and the outcome of your action. If you can only say "pain in abdomen" because you have no further assessment skills, it is appropriate to note what you did with the data. For example: "1030: c/o abdominal pain, consulted with assigned staff/instructor."

Subsequent notes should include a more experienced practitioner's assessment, evaluation, and action, with a follow-up recording the outcome of the intervention. You can compare this to writing a complete sentence: the patient complaint or observation is the subject, the intervention or action is the verb, and the outcome represents the object.

You are beginning to see how your note paints a complete picture of the patient and of individual practice standards. This picture is fixed in time. The charted time must reflect the time of patient contact even if you are not actually writing in the chart until the end of the day. Your note describes your observations and assessment based on your current level of expertise. It reflects what you did about the problem, your actions, both assessment measures and interventions. The outcome is noted. Did the intervention make a difference? What was the patient's response? Are further interventions necessary? Did you follow up appropriately and in a timely manner?

If your documentation does not include all the components for complete and precise charting, your notation is incomplete. Subsequent caregivers will not know if an intervention was done or if it worked.

If there are no complaints, this is also noteworthy. Contact with the patient must be documented. The documented time spent with individual patients verifies that they have had caregiver attention on each shift; it is the map used in recreating the progress of a patient's hospital visit. It is also important in assigning nursing hours to that patient, and to patients with similar needs, and ensuring that they are in the appropriate unit based on necessary hours of care.

The patient can state that he is "fine" and the nurse's eyes and senses may detect a problem. Facial expressions and body language are clues to be read and assessed further. If a patient denies pain while grimacing with movement and holding their breath as they move ever so slowly, the nurse uses assessment tools to support the observation of "suspected pain." Facies pain scales, most often used with children, along with measurement of vital signs can objectively support an observation.

Answer Guide

Exercise 2.1

1. arrest
   Common: seize and hold under legal authority
   Technical: stopped, as in organ function or disease process

2. mole
   Common: small mammal; undercover spy
   Technical: small, raised growth on skin; intrauterine mass

3. appreciate
   Common: think well of or value
   Technical: recognize quality of symptom

4. contraction
   Common: shortened word form
   Technical: muscle shortening or an increase in tension; heartbeat; expulsive muscle shortening during labor

5. hardware
   Common: articles made of metal; tools; parts of a computer
   Technical: orthopedic appliances for internal or external use

6. eliminate
   Common: get rid of; to remove
   Technical: expel waste material from body

7. evacuate
   Common: withdraw from a hazardous place; vacate
   Technical: empty, especially bowel waste; remove from, as with uterine contents

8. articulate
   Common:well-spoken
   Technical: jointed; surface meeting of joints

9. accommodate
   Common: willing to do a favor; lodging; a convenience
   Technical: state of adjustment or adaptation especially eye focus

10. appendix
    Common: supplemental section at end of book
    Technical: an appendage, most commonly related to the small bowel

11. humor
    Common: ability to be funny, comic
    Technical: fluid or semifluid substance in body

12. artifact
    Common: man-made object, often of historical interest
    Technical: anything caused incidentally by technique used rather than natural occurrence

13. excitement
    Common: elicit, provoke
    Technical: potential for stimulation

14. accessory
    Common: something extra but nonessential; someone who helps another break laws
    Technical: auxiliary, as with muscles or nerves

15. bed
    Common: sleeping furniture; ground for planting
    Technical: supporting structure for tissue

16. beat
    Common: hit repeatedly; surpass or defeat
    Technical: stroke or pulsation

17. capture
    Common: seize or take possession of by force; represent
    Technical: normal response of heart muscle to electrical impulse

18. crown
    Common: ornament; coin; hit or strike on head
    Technical: top or highest part of organ; presentation of baby's head in birth canal; dental prosthesis

19. dress
    Common: to put on clothes; one-piece style of woman's apparel
    Technical: apply cover to support or protect wound

20. drain
    Common: draw off liquid; channel or pipe; to empty
    Technical: tube to remove discharge or fluid from cavity

21. retention
    Common: hold, keep possession of; to hire
    Technical: keeping body waste normally, as with urine retention

22. bag
    Common: flexible container; to grab or capture; area of interest
    Technical: pouch or container to hold and/or measure body fluids or drainage

23. papoose
    Common: Native American infant
    Technical: method for restraining a child for a procedure

24. line
    Common: narrow continuous mark; boundary; covering for an interior surface
    Technical: access cannula for vascular testing or medicating

25. standing
    Common: positioned upright
    Technical: prepared instructions to be performed automatically under specific conditions

26. amplitude
    Common: great size; fullness
    Technical: measure of an action potential

27. conduction
    Common: to lead; to transmit
    Technical: transmission of energy from one point to another

28. discharge
    Common: relieve of a burden or task; to fire from a job
    Technical: secretion or excretion of a body fluid; release from care

29. labor
    Common: work or task; those who do work for others for wages
    Technical: effort expended for activity as breathing; process of delivering fetus

30. irrigation
    Common: to water, artificially
    Technical: to wash wound with saline or medicated fluids

Exercise 2.2

1. G; 2. E; 3. O; 4. H; 5. R; 6. I; 7. B; 8. L; 9. A; 10. C; 11. S;
12. P; 13. J; 14. K; 15. Q; 16. D; 17. M; 18. F; 19. N

Exercise 2.3

1. **Transpose new bag of solution:** take down the current IV solution bag and replace it with the next, new bag of IV solution to be infused
   Existing line: the IV in place
   Run at 100/hour: the drip is to be infused at the rate of 100 cc per hour

2. **Measure the patient's I & O:** monitor and measure either directly or if necessary by estimation the oral and parenteral fluids taken in by the patient as well as measuring urinary output
   Force fluids: increase the patient's fluid intake
   Output less than 50 cc/hour: average urination or "voiding" is less than 50 cc each hour

3. **Titrate:** regulate the flow of IV drip fluids or medication
   Maintain: to keep steady
   BP@90 systolic: top number of blood pressure no less than 90 mm Hg

4. **Turn:** move patient side to side
   Cough and deep breathe: take three deep breaths inward and expel the last deep breath in the form of a cough
   q 2h: every two hours

5. **Adjust O2 from 1 L:** the nurse will change the oxygen delivery system, which is set at 1 liter, an increased level of O2 than exists in a normal environment
Room air: the mixture of gases that usually exists in a normal room environment
15 min q hr: for 15 minutes of each hour

6. **NPO:** acronym for "nothing by mouth" or withhold food and fluids
Supine: positioned flat on back
Spinal study: any test in which the patient's spinal column is accessed

Exercise 2.4

1. "**He** didn't hear what I said."
"He **didn't** hear what I said."
"He didn't **hear** what I said."
"He didn't hear **what** I said."
"He didn't hear what **I** said."
"He didn't hear what I **said**."

2. "**You** can't try that with me."
"You **can't** try that with me."
"You can't **try** that with me."
"You can't try **that** with me."
"You can't try that **with** me."
"You can't try that with **me**."

3. "**Will** you stop and listen to me?"
"Will **you** stop and listen to me?"
"Will you **stop** and listen to me?"
"Will you stop **and** listen to me?"
"Will you stop and **listen** to me?"
"Will you stop and listen **to me**?"

4. "**Everything** he did seemed to make things better."
"Everything **he** did seemed to make things better."
"Everything he **did** seemed to make things better."
"Everything he did **seemed** to make things better."
"Everything he did seemed to make **things** better."
"Everything he did seemed to make things **better**."

5. "**You** never listen to what I say."
"You **never** listen to what I say."
"You never **listen** to what I say."
"You never listen to **what** I say."
"You never listen to what **I** say."
"You never listen to what I **say**."

Exercise 2.5

1. Statement: "pt. slept through noc"
Intention: According to the caregiver, the patient slept for the entire night without event or difficulty.
Legal Validity: An attempt to document a routine and, presumably, an uneventful night in which we are told the patient slept. However, there are no pertinent or objective observations or assessments in the statement that would support the entry if reviewed. The caregiver would be questioned as to how he or she was able to determine whether the patient was sleeping, and if in fact closed eyes or unlabored respirations meant the patient was actually asleep. If so, was the caregiver at the bedside of the patient the entire night? How would the caregiver possibly be in a position to know any physical

findings verifying that the patient slept throughout the night without waking, even once.

Professional Discrimination: The caregiver is making an effort to document the patient's status throughout the night during which he or she was responsible for providing safety and care needs to the patient. It is desirable, and oftentimes an actuality, that patients sleep well and for the duration of the night. This example, however, provides a purely subjective statement as to what the caregiver determined to be the patient's physical state of rest. It is much more useful for the caregiver to describe objective assessments that may be related to the subjective judgment "slept all night." Even so, statements such as "eyes closed," "respirations quiet and unlabored," "offered no complaints," "appeared to rest when checked hourly" would not in fact equate with sleep. It is better to avoid drawing conclusions from subjectively based presumptions. Simply note the physical markers for the patient's relatively stable or unchanging status and let the objective assessment stand its own.

2. Statement: "complains of slight pain with palpation"
    Intent: The patient reported or confirmed insignificant or unsubstantial pain upon palpation.
    Legal Validity: Document an amount of pain expressed by the patient upon palpation. However, the notation is vague in that it does not reflect where the palpation and subsequent pain occurred. There is an attempt to quantify the amount of pain by using a broad generalization, slight, in the entry, which does not leave the reader with any specific indicator as to where the pain was located or how much palpation elicited how much pain. Additionally, the word used to describe the quantity of pain is not entered in quotation marks and presumably is purely the caregiver's determination of how substantial the pain was to the patient.
    Professional Discrimination: It is vital to include documentation of the patient's sense of pain. However, you must avoid suppositions when attempting to describe how much pain the patient sustained. It is extremely important to note the exact location, intensity, and duration of the pain. The nurse does not feel the pain; it is a completely subjective patient response and varies enormously from patient to patient. Even in the presence of a consistent stimulus, individual patients relate different experiences with pain. Your responsibility is to objectively assess and determine the extent of the pain. Often a nurse may use some measurement system to describe the amount of pain felt. If such a system is being used, it is important to let the patient's own subjective measurement be the actual determination. Words or numbers a patient would assign to pain should always be in quotation marks.

3. Statement: "tolerated procedure well"
    Intent: The caregiver is describing that the patient managed the procedure without difficulty.
    Legal Validity: This is a supposition of the part of the nurse. There is an effort to note how the patient fared during a procedure; however, there are no objective assessments supporting the statement. Without some physical evidence relative to the patient's status and procedure measured by the caregiver, no evidence supports the determination. Of course, direct statements from the patient in quotation marks are always accurate and appropriate representations of the patient's status.
    Professional Discrimination: It is very important to document a patient's status during an invasive, therapeutic, or diagnostic procedure. Once again, however, your entry must have a quantifiable basis and meaning to maintain validity. The absence of quotation marks on the word tolerated indicates that it was the

nurse's subjective observation as to how the patient did during the procedure. You may draw conclusions on a limited basis; however, any presumptions must be fully upheld with factual assessments. Without objective, supportive measurements, the basis for presumption does not exist.

4. Statement: "appears in no distress"
Intent: The patient was not experiencing physical discomfort or emotional anxiety.
Legal Validity: This is a conclusion on the part of the caregiver. There are no additional notations or statements in quotation marks to provide evidence or support as to how the patient felt. The caregiver has presumed (from his or her personal vantage point) the patient's amount of stress.
Professional Discrimination: Unfortunately, there is a decided lack of tangible assessments or measures to support the conclusion stated by the nurse. It is important to note a patient's level of distress, especially in the presence of a change or new symptom. However, to do so in subjective terms, and without indications that the words used are directly from the patient renders the entry inaccurate and groundless.

5. Statement: "resting comfortably when checked hourly"
Intent: A statement of the patient's state of well-being and level of distress on an hourly basis. This in an effort to indicate that the patient was being checked on at least hourly and without any sudden or precipitous change in status.
Legal Validity: For patients in a chronic, long-term, or stabilized care environment, there is the legal responsibility to make at least an hourly check of the patient's status. Depending upon the institutional setting, a patient's condition may not change for weeks, months, or even years. The responsibility to verify that the patient's state remains stable is frequently noted in the nursing documentation on an hourly basis. Generally an hourly notation is associated with a patient in a subacute setting rather than a long-term or institutionalized setting. An existing standard, however, is that the patient's condition be reviewed by a caregiver on (at least) an hourly basis.
Professional Discrimination: The statement is intended to reflect that the patient was both checked hourly and remained stable without acute change. As an entry into the nursing record, there are no indicators to reinforce the caregiver's subjective determination of *resting* or *comfortably*. Without further objective assessments (i.e., of vital signs or pain measurements), the notation has no basis for support and would easily be disqualified.

Exercise 2.6

1. catheter
2. IV catheter
3. cardiac catheter
4. urinary catheter
5. anterior
6. dilate
7. junction
8. joint
9. stopcock
10. fundus
11. obtunded
12. dress

13. local
14. stream
15. radiation

Exercise 2.7

1. The nurse adjusted the dial setting to increase the visual display representing the electrical impulses in a patient's cardiac cycle.
2. The nurse instructed the patient prior to the patient's leaving the hospital additional precautions when either voiding directly or if emptying a catheter device inserted into the patient's urinary bladder.
3. The patient gave his or her signature agreeing to an orthopedic operation to repair a fracture or a bone with or without implanted hardware to stabilize the bone ends somewhere in the body.
4. If a patient left the direct care and supervision of his or her physician and nurses, there may be legal consequences because the patient was no longer under the direct care of a medical professional.
5. There was an apparent mechanism for injury to the eyeball but that the circular, contained body of the eye was intact and the liquid contained therein was not disturbed.
6. A wound that the patient sustained was healing, and there was evidence that new tissue was being regenerated.
7. A member of the health care team had been unable to use the cardiac monitor record to screen an image of a peculiar or abnormal cardiac cycle of concern to the physician.

Exercise 2.8

1. arrest
2. reduction
3. exquisite
4. accessory
5. accommodation
6. radiated
7. conduction
8. fundus
9. atrophy
10. catheter
11. crown
12. eliminate
13. standing orders
14. papoose
15. pattern

Exercise 2.9

1. What area of the abdomen does the patient call their "stomach" (location)? What does "hurt" mean to the patient (quality and quantity of pain, chronology, setting, associated manifestations, alleviating/aggravating factors)?

2. Where does the patient's head hurt? Is this an expected effect of a procedure? Is it related to the admitting diagnosis?

3. In what position is the patient (supine, sitting)? Is the patient unable move or is there another factor involved? Could the patient "get up" and around before this moment?

4. What does the patient mean by "dizzy"? Would the patient's condition or medication cause this feeling? What was the patient doing when they began to feel dizzy?

5. To what sensation is the patient referring? What position makes the patient's feet "feel funny"? Has the patient had a medication or procedure that might affect the sensation in the lower limbs?

Exercise 2.10

1. $>$ greater than
2. $<$ less than
3. $>$ greater than
4. $>$ greater than
5. $<$ less than
6. $>$ greater than
7. $<$ less than
8. $>$ greater than
9. $<$ less than

CHAPTER 3

Format Made Easy

WORD LIST

collateral	lacrimation	turn
lead	lactate	vapors
digit	pattern	coping
macerate	phalanx	void
nonresponsive	run	maintain
stool	flush	titrate
piggyback	lacerate	
patent	transpose	

 Exercise 3.1

Each item in the word list has both common and technical meanings. Match each word with its corresponding set of definitions and compare the intent or usage of the terms as both common and technical words.

1. _____
   Common: corroborating, supporting, indirect
   Technical: subsidiary to primary, as with arteries

2. _____
   Common: top of wall
   Technical: ability to face problem and resolve it

3. _____
   Common: number
   Technical: finger or toe

4. _____
   Common: to flow copiously; to blush or turn red; poker hand with cards all in the same suit; hunting term for exposing game birds; to wash out a toilet with copious amounts of water
   Technical: to irrigate or wash out with large amounts of water

5. _____
   Common: rip; tear
   Technical: tear tissue; wound with jagged edge

6. _____
   Common: secretion of tears
   Technical: tears

7. _____
   Common: to secrete milk
   Technical: a product of lactic acid; to produce milk

8. _____
   Common: to guide or direct; to be at head; dull gray metal
   Technical: connection for electrical conduction usually between a patient and measuring device

9. _____
   Common: to soak in liquid to soften and separate into components
   Technical: to soften or make thin

10. _____
    Common: to continue; to keep in good condition
    Technical: to comply with good health practice

11. _____
    Common: to not reply, not react
    Technical: no reaction, physical or mental, to applied stimulus

12. _____
    Common: government document that ensures inventor's rights; obvious
    Technical: opened, not plugged

13. _____
    Common: A tightly grouped formation
    Technical: singular for long bones of fingers

14. _____
    Common: term for one person carrying another on shoulders; truck trailer carried on the flat car of train
    Technical: to deliver a bag of IV solution by injecting into existing IV tubing

15. _____
    Common: to move rapidly on foot; to compete for an elected office; to drive or steer
    Technical: to deliver fluids or medications through IV

16. _____
    Common: seat with no back or arms; footrest
    Technical: fecal material

17. _____
    Common: determine solution concentration
    Technical: deliver solution in a specific concentration over a defined time period

18. _____
    Common: to change or reverse the order of
    Technical: to replace existing IV fluid bag with a new or different bag; to change placement of organs or tissue

19. _____
    Common: move or cause to move
    Technical: change patient position on a regular schedule

20. _____

    Common: gaseous state of a normally liquid or solid matter; old-fashioned term for feeling poorly

    Technical: inhaled medication

21. _____

    Common: empty; unoccupied

    Technical: to urinate or defecate

22. _____

    Common: design or model; routine way of doing things

    Technical: recognizable model; repetitive behavior trait

DOCUMENTATION FORMAT

A system for organizing words that facilitates reader comprehension is known as a format. Words such as form, formal, deformed, and formula are derived from the same Latin root word, *forma*. This chapter focuses your learning on how to arrange, how to format, your documentation. Your goal is to develop an organized system in which to record assessments and related patient priorities. Your written report should provide clarity to subsequent caregivers while complying with the standards of your facility. Later on, in Chapters 6 and 7, you will practice using your own system, your format, while working with sample clinical case studies.

A health care facility creates many of its own documentation forms and requires measurable and manageable uniformity from its staff. It is a responsibility of the risk management department to review forms for completeness; however, it is your responsibility to "fill in the blanks" of the patient care you delivered. You must be sure you have concisely transcribed all information necessary to reflect safe and legal patient care. Include all information that may describe or affect patient outcomes. Because there is "no place to write it" is not an acceptable reason to omit relevant patient data.

As a nurse, you are expected to know what information is necessary to include. As a student, you are busy learning how to perform the technical tasks of nursing and not necessarily associating how to organize or remember information you may have obtained doing the task. How does one learn to discriminate, not just between words, but between entire information sets?

A practical method to organize your written or verbal communication while learning to discriminate within patient information sets is to choose a style or format at the beginning of your nursing education. Work to improve your skills as you develop and increase your vocabulary. The combination of learning technical words while you are manually performing an associated task helps you to differentiate and classify data and shows you how to collect information you will later use to complete your patient's record. Each health care facility has unique requirements; the format you select must be adaptable.

This workbook focuses on the Complete Health History (CHH) and the physical exam (PE). These formats are commonly accepted in medical education and variations are located in many medical-surgical nursing textbooks. CHH and PE are commonly used methods found in the dictated histories of many patient records. The organized style has evolved through practice to include the trend toward treating the whole patient, to address the holistic influences in medicine. The CHH and PE formats include specific and detailed information, organized and documented in a manner that assists the care provider to differentiate and follow individualized, yet appropriate treatment paths. Reimbursement laws require that precise and exact details of the patient status be documented. Chapter 8 of this workbook elaborates upon medical and legal considerations that indicate the desirability of a formatted style of documentation.

> ### BOX 3.1
> # Problem-Oriented Charting
>
> Problem-oriented charting is focused on a specific problem or complaint. It is primarily used after a CHH has been completed, and is incorporated into a patient record. It is also used by "drop in" clinics that do not focus on primary care. In problem-oriented charting, the interviewer solicits information necessary to provide immediate attention for a specific complaint.
>
> This interview may be conducted using a "menu," wherein unlicensed personnel ask the patient to complete a check list and/or answer a limited number of questions. The provider then examines the patient, and documents his or her physical findings in the chart. The provider then writes the treatment given or ordered (Rx) with the discharge note or disposition of the patient.
>
> Nurses working in these settings who are doing procedures and giving injections need to "double check" on the data that may be critical to patient care. Key areas to recheck are allergies, current medications, immunizations, and exposures.

THE COMPLETE HEALTH HISTORY (CHH)

The format style for the CHH and PE determines the order of presentation. If modified to present chief complaint, it is often referred to as "problem-oriented charting," wherein the critical event is represented and followed by comorbid factors in order of relevance to the primary complaint. If associated problems are determined to be equally weighted, use the order inherent to the CHH and PE. Health professionals are familiar with the format's style and depend upon its organization to receive and process information about the patient's health status. The uniformity of the format promotes consistency of care standards among different providers.

As you begin to function in a clinical setting, you will understand the importance of choosing and developing an organized system for assessment and documentation. Incorporating newly learned technical language into your documentation format will help establish a pattern. This in turn will enhance your nurse process and time management skills. You will be able to recall information more readily and the organized format of the CHH and PE will assert a positive influence on your assessment techniques as well.

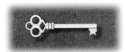

By developing a standardized format, consistently applied, you will minimize the risk for errors based upon omission. You will learn to use language to document specific or significant elements. Your selected use of language, in combination with a "head to toe" order, prioritizing data and using objective parameters is, in itself, a format style. The uniformity found in the CHH and PE will permit you to create a sense of style and organization in your documentation that should mean the same the day you enter your nursing career as on the day you conclude it. The fluid and dynamic nature of medicine and health care requires you to develop a method that establishes consistency yet allows flexibility.

Given the potential for physical, medical, or legal consequences, it would seem that a logical and organized progression of documentation, with connected descriptors throughout the note, would be instinctive. This is not necessarily the case with all students and may well reflect the lack of association between language and tasks. As a student is learning nursing tasks, the focus is on hand skills rather than emphasis on assessment or documentation.

Quite naturally a student is more absorbed in how the needle is entering the patient rather than the language describing the precise anatomical point of entry or the receptivity of the tissue once the needle penetrates the skin surface.

This is what makes CHH and PE so valuable. In themselves, they represent a system of organization that directs your description of patient care events. As you become more proficient with language use, your charting system will include and reflect pertinent events and appropriate care.

Now let's get an introduction to and begin to practice with the CHH and PE. The CHH is generally obtained by the primary care provider. As a bedside, clinical nurse you may well be the interviewer who obtains and records this information. Your nursing objectives are to learn how to document, how to review a written history, and how to use the information contained within the history in the care of your patients.

Pay careful attention to avoid misspellings, transcription errors, or misinformation in the patient's record. Avoid transcribing subjective, patient-based information in anything other than quotation marks. Misunderstandings and errors are possible and often occur with the information transfer process. Read your documentation to determine if it clearly states what you meant.

The following is an introduction to the CHH. You can practice the CHH interview with another student or family and friends. Remember as we review the elements of the CHH that patient information is always confidential!

INFORMANT

The informant is the person who is giving the information. It does not refer to someone you might associate with selling information in a darkened alleyway. The informant can be anyone, but is most often the patient (Box 3.2), a relative of the patient, a friend, or even a bystander.

BOX 3.2

Informant

Any person, usually the patient, who is cooperative and can give reliable information.

PATIENT PROFILE

The Patient Profile is designed to be an objective and broadly inclusive account of who the patient is. Generally included is the patient's name, age, sex, race or ethnic heritage, marital status, occupation, and in some cases, a diagnosis or presenting problem and who referred the patient to the facility or office. Race and ethnicity are not exactly the same thing and differences between the two may affect lab

---

BOX 3.3

Patient Profile

Patient Profile: Mr. M. is a 33 year old male, a single, Hispanic, unemployed refugee from El Salvador, referred from Occupational Health Clinic with a positive PPD.
Or
Patient Profile: Mr. M., 33 yo, Hisp., M, S, unemployed, refugee from El Salvador, referred from Occupational Health Clinic c̄ +PPD.

BOX 3.4

Culture and Age

Race, culture, ethnicity, and gender often contribute to the diagnosis or treatment of a patient. Studies conducted on certain disease pathologies highlight the frequency of occurrence along racial and ethnic lines. Studies of drugs include a drug's efficacy among gender and race. The provider's choice of drug treatment may well be based on the results of these studies. It is reasonable to include culture and ethnicity in the patient profile.

Be as accurate as possible when recording the profile. Remember that when you record this information it is not to "classify" the patient but to provide information to enhance care.

Age is an objective number. Race, ethnicity, and culture can be more controversial, and it may be difficult to determine in which category a patient may fit. If you are uncertain of a patient's race and/or ethnicity, always ask. For example, a dark-skinned individual may be profiled as African-American, though neither African nor American. A native Hawaiian may be profiled as Asian. As you can see this can be confusing at best and inaccurate and harmful as well.

Use the guidelines approved by your practice setting in recording this information. Remember that there are basically four recognized races but many ethnic variations. A person's cultural habits may not necessarily reflect their ethnic heritage.

work ordered, which medications are given, and discharge teaching plan. Does this sound like a lot of data to include? Box 3.3 is an example for you to consider.

Practice charting these data first as a "list." Seeing the information as separate bits of information can help you to remember what is necessary for the chart as well as how to organize the data.

Identify the patient: Mr. M. (Identifying the patient by name clarifies who you are describing, personalizes the report, and helps to keep the patient from being thought of as a disease or injury. It is respectful.)

Age: 33 yo (Age information further describes the patient as well as defining the medical risk group to which he belongs. Risk prevention and health protection rely on the providers' being aware of these risk groups in order to provide appropriate health teaching.)

Race/ethnicity: Hisp. (Race adds to information necessary for risk assessment and for health teaching. It is also pertinent in screening and in prescribing medications. Placement of race prior to gender is descriptive rather than prioritization: it creates a picture of the patient being described.)

Gender: M (see "Race/ethnicity")

Marital status: S (This information gives the provider data regarding the patient's support system and about responsibilities that may be affected by hospital confinement. Status of parenthood may or may not be included. This is a judgment decision based on if the hospitalized or sick parent will have significant added stress while separated from the family or if there is significant impact on complaint or care path.)

Employment status: Church employee (Relates to patient's responsibilities that will be affected as well as his ability to pay for care.)

Pertinent personal/social data: refugee from El Salvador (Relates to potential risk factors, as well as other stressors which may affect care. It may also give cultural information regarding the patient's response to isolation.)

Patient of or referral source: referred from Occupational Health Clinic (Current caregivers need access to health information. With some diseases, like tuberculosis (TB), it is necessary to know whether symptoms caused the disease to be diagnosed or if it was routine screening.)

Reason for referral/complaint: +PPD (Screening related to employment revealed a positive PPD. Refugee status from a country that has a high incidence of TB becomes pertinent data. Living and working environments are also important due to potential exposure.)

BOX 3.5

Essential Patient Profile Data

ID:
Age:
Race:
Marital status:
Employment status:
Pt. of/referral/or complaint:

The Complete Health History will contain far more information and details than your admitting history in hospital. You will have a CHH or History and Physical from the admitting provider in the chart. It is up to you to use judgment in your admitting history.

For example, would a patient be admitted to isolation for a +PPD alone? Probably not. There was probably a follow-up chest X-ray (CXR) that added to the suspicion of active TB. The hospitalization would be to isolate the patient, preventing the possibility of further exposing the general public to TB. Your hospital admission history might then state "admitted for +PPD, +CXR, R/O [rule out] TB."

You will use discretion and judgment in deciding the pieces of information necessary for your history and for all additional nursing notes. Identifying the patient is not necessary for each note; it is necessary for each newly instigated verbal report to other caregivers. Once the patient is identified the caregivers familiar with the patient most likely will visualize the patient from his or her admitting profile. If not, you can refresh the provider's memory by restating the profile.

If the patient information is not essential to the patient profile, it may be appropriate in another section. For instance, data regarding a patient's family, especially if it is about older well children, need not be in the patient profile but might better be related in the personal/social history section. Situational life stresses and support systems are part of each patient's experiential learning that affects their response to medical care.

 Exercise 3.2

In the following exercise, practice charting patient profile data. Remember to include ID, age, race, marital status, employment status, and patient of/referral/or complaint in your answer.

1. Patient A
   Your patient is a 55-year-old man who is black. He tells you he lives with his wife and still has one 17-year-old child living at home. He has retired from the navy but is self-employed doing tractor work. He was admitted for left inguinal hernia repair.

   _____

   _____

   _____

2. Patient B
   Your assignment is to interview a patient of Dr. ABC who was admitted for right-sided heart failure. The patient is an 80-year-old female whose husband died three months ago. She is white and has 5 children, 3 of whom are still living.

   _____

   _____

   _____

3. Patient C
   You are admitting a 17-year-old Asian who found a pea-sized lump in his scrotum and has a possible tumor on his right testicle. He is due to graduate from high school in five months. He lives with his parents and one younger sister.

   _____

   _____

   _____

4. Patient D
   You are assigned the patient in Room 413. She is white, age 35, who is admitted with a lump in her left breast. Her husband and two preschool-aged children are in the room when you arrive. Her husband wears a yarmulke, and they are praying.

   _____

   _____

   _____

5. Patient E
   Your patient is a 5-month-old girl admitted for respiratory dysfunction. She was brought in by her sister who watches her while her parents work. The sister is monolingual in Mandarin Chinese and is accompanied by an aunt who acts as an interpreter.

   _____

   _____

   _____

CHIEF COMPLAINT

The chief complaint is most often entered in the note in quotation marks. It is commonly identified as the reason the patient gave as to why they believe they need medical attention (Box 3.6). It is relevant to the current visit to the physician, the emergency department, or clinic rather than any earlier visit, even if for the same complaint or symptoms. This is a subjective element and is usually not amended by the interviewer. If the patient is not the informant (see Box 3.2) it should be so noted. Similarly if a translator is being used, that must also be documented. If you are working in a setting which uses a SOAP format, the chief complaint is noted under "S" (subjective). It is a challenge to be brief yet accurate when relating the chief complaint. Oftentimes patients with complicated medical histories will provide much more information than the precise reason

BOX 3.6

Chief Complaint

"I might have TB."

> ### BOX 3.7
>
> ## SOAP Format
>
> Many clinics and home health agency's use a charting format known as SOAP, an acronym for subjective, objective, assessment, plan. This format helps the provider include data required for accreditation review and for reimbursement.
>
> The subjective note records the problem in the patient's own words. It is usually a direct patient statement of the immediate problem which has compelled the patient to seek assistance.
>
> The objective data include the provider's quantitative observations. Data are presented in a logical manner and often include vital signs, physical assessment, and lab results. Psychosocial observations, for example an observation of restlessness, would be charted as mannerisms of the patient's supported by indicators such as eye movement, position shifting, or pacing.
>
> The assessment is a concluding statement that clearly indicates what the nurse or other provider believes is the problem or cluster of problems. The assessment is based on the objective information available at the time.
>
> The plan includes diagnostic tests, referrals, immediate treatment recommendations, and disposition of the patient. It should also include what the provider of care will do to follow up, or evaluate, the outcome of any planned intervention.

for seeking medical attention that particular day. As the interviewer, it is your responsibility to discriminate between information points and to record the patient's exact reason for accessing health care at the time of this visit or hospital admission.

 ## Exercise 3.3

In this simple exercise you will determine which statement represents the patient's chief complaint. A clue: The chief complaint is always a direct quote by the patient.

 Example:

    a. "I woke up and felt very hot and sweaty."
    b. Patient woke up feeling feverish.

    The answer is "a."

1. a. Patient c/o backache
   b. "My back hurts when I sit down"
2. a. Decreased visual acuity
   b. "I feel like I am looking through a dirty window"
3. a. Possible appendicitis
   b. "I have bad stomach cramps and feel like throwing up"
4. a. Fractured femur
   b. "I broke my leg playing touch football"
5. a. "I have a cold and my nose is stuffy"
   b. Upper respiratory infection

HISTORY OF PRESENT ILLNESS

At this time, the interviewer will investigate the patient's chief complaint. One commonly used method, essentially a format within a format, is used throughout this workbook. You will be investigating the patient's presenting history using descriptors (Box 3.8); that is, you will use language tools to ascertain symptom type, location, quality, quantity, timing, setting, aggravating or alleviating factors, associated manifestations, and the meaning of the symptom to the patient. Committing the descriptor categories to memory is useful in all clinical areas. Information about the present illness is useful in the acute or primary care setting where nurses complete a history with supporting data, vital to planning patient care. Accuracy is a prerequisite to good patient care.

If you are in a setting using the SOAP format, the history of present illness is noted under "O" (objective).

BOX 3.8

History of Present Illness

Patient is feeling healthy but was transferred to hospital because of a positive test for tuberculosis, post one week employment. Loss of appetite accompanied by a 15 lb. weight loss, which he thought was due to "smoking cocaine." C/O occasional night sweats times 5 months, clear nasal drainage, and has felt warm but denies fever, cough, chest pain, dyspnea, hemoptysis, chills, fatigue, infections, or allergies and sensitivities. Positive history of drug use ("smoking cocaine"), 4 pack years cigarette smoking. PH positive for HBV 1988 (sexual contact), treated with no sequelae. FH noncontributory. OH negative for respiratory exposure. P/SH anxiety re: TB, incarceration, and disabled mate's daily care.

CONCURRENT HEALTH PROBLEMS

Concurrent health problems is a chronological listing of ongoing health issues not necessarily related to the patient's current complaint. You should include all acute and chronic health problems, although extensive descriptions are not usually necessary. It is pertinent to include onset, duration, and any present treatment of the stated health problem.

Objective data collection in this category can be challenging. Patients use their own words to characterize ailments. You will hear statements such as "I've got the blues" or "vapors" to describe depression and fatigue, and "medicine to thin my blood" for anticoagulant therapy. There may also be symptoms of a more private nature to the patient, who, upon questioning, may not even mention problems of sexual dysfunction or complaints involving the genitalia.

Your interview skills ideally will adapt to the emotional, physical, situational, and developmental needs of the patient. We use language to communicate verbally, but a large share of communication is done nonverbally as well. Think of an instance where you were unable to communicate a technical question to a patient. Was it with a non–English speaking patient, an elderly shut-in, or a small toddler? It is a challenge sometimes to communicate effectively. Using techniques or language that are patronizing, embarrassing to the patient, or which lead the patient to say things that are inaccurate must be consciously avoided.

BOX 3.9

First Impressions

Your use of language throughout the interview process will be instrumental in determining the quality of the interview. You will benefit by learning to make a quick assessment of your patient as you introduce yourself. Patients appreciate knowing to whom they are speaking, so always identify yourself and tell them your professional status. Tell them why you are there but don't ask for their approval. Even with student status, you are part of a health care team. It is not appropriate to end your introduction with "I'll be your nurse today, is that all right [or OK] with you?" It is appropriate for you to pause after the introduction to allow the patient to assess you.

Many cultures need a getting-to-know-you period that is difficult to accomplish within the time constraints of patient care. A short pause prior to continuing your interview offers the patient a moment to process your status. Some cultures "give you permission," spoken or unspoken, to continue. Consider this example: "Good Morning, I'm Joe, a student nurse, and I will be taking care of you today. How is your pain?" Hispanics, Native Americans, and some Asian groups may be reluctant to participate if you end your introduction with your first question.

After a pause, you may begin your questions, moving from broad to more discrete inquiries. If you are working on history taking, you might acknowledge that the patient may have been asked the same questions before (or the patient might believe you have come to the hospital totally unprepared). As you speak, assess the patient's ability to understand your language. Because a patient nods and appears to understand does not necessarily mean that this is the case. Adapt your language to the patient's level of understanding. If you ask when the patient last voided, they may say, "I don't know." You might get an accurate answer if you ask them when they last "peed."

Within selective settings such as the emergency department, staff may need to immediately ascertain information regarding emergent, critical health problems. This information is analogous to that under concurrent health problems in the CHH, but on a priority basis. A long-term history of diabetes in a comatose victim is likely to be more relevant in the precipitous condition than say, chronic back pain.

Verbal report to physicians and oncoming shifts is your opportunity to summarize patient data. Prioritization, organization, brevity, and relevancy are imperative to ensure accuracy and efficiency.

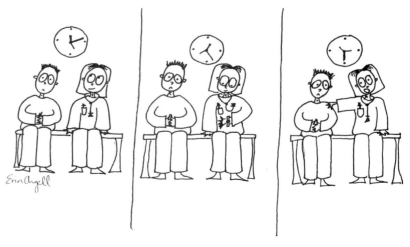

"You've gotta start the interview"

BOX 3.10

Focusing on Pertinent Details

Prioritization: You are learning how to prioritize patient data in class and in clinical. You will be integrating this knowledge into your charting and verbal report. Learn to differentiate between what is a critical nursing priority and what is the patient's perceived priority. Don't trivialize the patient's wishes but do be prepared for possible conflict.

Relevancy: You must be learn to determine the actual relevancy of your data. For instance, how many degrees of increased temperature are remarkable for a particular patient. Relevance is usually determined in relationship to a complete data set.

Organization: Keep data sets together. Unrelated bits of information scattered throughout a written or verbal report are likely to be overlooked. Cohesive information is far more likely to be interpreted as valuable data that may support a logical conclusion.

Brevity: Don't ramble on like a storyteller. Your audience, the members of the team caring for your patients, is working under time limitations. Clear concise data sharing is key. It may leave you time to share less critical information that is important in holistic management of patient needs.

Accuracy: Specific data must be accurate. Misinformation may result in error. If you are unsure of your data, check and recheck before it becomes part of a patient's chart. "I don't know, I will check" is a better response than a guess.

Efficiency: Use the correct words wisely. Complete information is more important here than complete sentences.

PAST HEALTH HISTORY

The past health history (PHH) narrates all known health-related events in the patient's life from birth to the present. It is an unembellished record that allows the current caregivers to view a snapshot of preventive care along with usual and remarkable medical events. This history is most often completed by the primary care provider. Often, practitioners use a check-off format to obtain this data. The checklist is a useful tool but is limited to broad categories, such as "cardiovascular disease." A personal interview, using language skills that help patients to recall details, is a more effective method of information exchange.

The PHH should contain clearly stated objective information (Box 3.11). Narrative lists are adequate for this overview. An exception is any event that oc-

---

BOX 3.11

Past Health History

A. Childhood
  1. Immunizations: polio and smallpox.
  2. Chicken pox, "dysentery" 1962 for which he was hospitalized for six months in El Salvador. Neg. rheumatic fever, measles, mumps, rubella, allergies.
B. Adulthood
  1. HBV (see HPI)
  2. Gonorrhea, 1988, treated with penicillin, no sequelae
  3. Fractured L radius, 1977, does not remember cause, no sequelae.
  4. Scabies infestation, 1990

C. Medications
  1. Tylenol (OTC)
  2. "pain killer" for toothache, 1993.
D. Allergies and sensitivities—none
E. Immunizations—see Childhood.
F. Additional Risk Data
  1. Nonoccupational exposure—drug use, incarceration
  2. PPD negative on immigration
  3. Health care providers—none
  4. Travel—Moved to Guerneville one month ago

BOX 3.11—*Continued*

Read the following example format and write your own health history.

A. Childhood
   1. Communicable diseases—list and date
   2. Illness/accidents/injuries—list, date, and describe as appropriate
   3. Surgery—list and date
   4. Immunizations—don't assume that parents have immunized their children
B. Adulthood
   1. Illness—chronic and acute
     a. Medical
     b. Occupational/litigation—discussing past or pending litigation with a patient requires skillful and nonjudgmental communication skills. Care needs to be taken to avoid trigger words that are demeaning to the patient.
   2. Surgery
   3. Accidents/injuries
   4. Psychiatric—medical-legal issues
   5. Allergies—Allergic reactions may not be remembered events. If the patient recalls no allergies it is better to record "none known" or "none stated."
   6. Medications
     a. Rx—In this context "Rx" represents prescription medications.
     b. OTC—abbreviation for "over the counter"
   7. Immunizations—Adult patients may not link the word immunization with a tetanus booster.
   8. Screening/prevention

The words "screening" and "prevention" are not necessarily common words to nonmedical persons. Screening clinics for vision and scoliosis are often held in schools. Screening for pregnancy may be a prerequisite for women over 12 years of age who need specific medications or who are seeking employment in hazardous areas. The words you use to solicit this information must be understandable to the general population.

"Prevention" is often thought of only in reference to preventive medications such as daily asthma medications or birth control pills. In the general population the word "prevention" may be thought of in the context of sexually transmitted disease or pregnancy. It is your job to ask about tuberculosis screening and prophylaxis, mammography, cholesterol screening, glaucoma tests, immunizations related to overseas travel, as these are less likely to be recalled by your patient.

When you interview for a CHH, understanding the global nature of the words "screening and prevention" will help you to use language that assists the patient to recall more data.

     a. PPD—date of last test. You may have to describe the testing process in order for an individual to know what a PPD or TB test is.
     b. Mammography
     c. Other
   9. Dental
  10. Eye—include a question about glasses; refraction is not always considered "eye problems."
  11. Additional risk factors—A patient might be uncomfortable when asked if they have any "risk factors" in their past or present that may contribute to their health status. In reality travel may be a direct link to diagnosis. Hobbies may also be contributors. Most people would not disclose the hobby of painting as a "risk factor" but this information may be key in treating a patient with cardiopulmonary symptoms.
     a. Travel—international travel is emphasized but all travel should be included in this section.
     b. Transfusions
     c. Exposures/hobbies
     d. Other

curred in the past that continues to affect the patient in the present. This is also true for disease that may no longer be an active problem but may contribute to understanding a patient's precipitating condition.

The PHH needs to be noted clearly and with nonjudgmental language. It is difficult for patients to discuss certain issues such as occupational injuries that may have resulted in litigation and disability. A problematic sexual history may be even more difficult to obtain. As you interview the patient, your body language is important and your choice of words must be age appropriate and culturally sensitive.

FAMILY HISTORY

The family history (FH) is usually noted as a list (Box 3.12). This is a section that may read: "Positive for diabetes, cardiovascular disease, and hypertension" in a narrative format or "+NIDDM, CVD, HTN" in an abbreviated style.

Diseases usually included in this category are CAD, HTN, CVD, DM, TB, CA, Migraine HA, seizures, colitis, renal, asthma, arthritis, obesity, and psychiatric disorders.

BOX 3.12

Family History

Mother—Headaches
Father—ETOH abuse, cough, liver disease
Brother—"heart attack" post injury age 22, negative family history of HTN, CVD, arthritis, gout, obesity, heart disease, diabetes, anemia, ulcer disease, TB, epilepsy, renal disease, psychiatric problems, or occupational exposure.

Exercise 3.4

Can you match the pathologies listed by initials with their spelled out form?

1.	CAD	cancer
2.	HTN	diabetes mellitus
3.	CVD	cardiovascular disease
4.	DM	hypertension
5.	TB	headache
6.	CA	tuberculosis
7.	HA	coronary artery disease

OCCUPATIONAL/ENVIRONMENTAL HISTORY

This entry includes the patient's work history, military service, potential, past/current exposures, injuries, hobbies, and environmental concerns (Box 3.13).

BOX 3.13

Occupational History

A. Past employment—1980: Restaurant work, dishwashing, janitorial
B. Current employment—Catholic Church handyman
C. Military employment—none

PERSONAL/SOCIAL HISTORY

The Personal/Social History (PSH) (Box 3.14) completes the picture of the whole patient. It allows the caregiver a glimpse into the patient's life as a complete person.

A. Family and cultural influences
B. Education
C. Marital/relationship history
D. Current life situation

BOX 3.14

Personal/Social History

A. Familial and Cultural Influences
Mr. F was born in a small village in El Salvador on May 28, 1960. He states his birth date was changed to May 4 for reason unknown to him. His family lived in two rooms and were "very poor." He is unsure of how his older brother died and was not born at the time it occurred. He does not know the ages of his surviving siblings but believes they are all in good health and in El Salvador. He states that he feels very fond of his family but has not returned to El Salvador because he has no money to bring to them. He is Roman Catholic, attends church and has good, positive feelings toward his religion. He states that his mother is well and still "works very hard" and that his siblings all live near her. He has one aunt who lives in Washington State, with whom he has no contact. Mr. F was granted asylum in the U.S. after illegal entry into Texas when he was 17. He moved to California in his early 20s when he agreed to drive a car to Utah for an acquaintance and was abandoned there without payment.

B. Education
Mr. F lived with his parents in El Salvador prior to immigration. He states the family was very poor, but that he has good memories of his family and his childhood. He attended Catholic school until about 7th grade and was taught by Franciscan priests. He came to the U.S. with a friend who was deported, but he was allowed to remain. He attended high school for a short period in Texas. He speaks English well and has some reading and writing skills in both English and Spanish.

C. Marital/Relationship History
Mr. F demonstrates a genuine affection for his housemate but his relationship with her is un-clear. He has no other significant relationships, has never been married, and has no children. He is concerned about the expense of care for his friend while he is in the hospital and is anxious about being gone for a long period of time. He has one other friend, male, in SC. He maintains no contact with friends from childhood.

D. Current Life Situation
Patient is single and lives with a woman who is disabled due to childhood polio. He performs household tasks, cooks, assists her with ADLs and mobility in exchange for room and board. She is confined to a wheelchair so he gets most of his exercise by providing physical assistance to her. He has no other exercise program except the physical demands of his job. He has no medical insurance. They have moved within the last month and he was in the Occupational Health Clinic for an employment physical, which resulted in hospitalization in the isolation unit.

E. Health Habits
   1. Nutrition—Prepares 3 meals/day, barbecues meat, vegetables, and starch regularly in diet. See appetite—HPI.
   2. Alcohol (ETOH) use—1–2 6 packs beer qd
   3. Smoking—see HPI
   4. Sleep—6–8 hours/night, see HPI
   5. Exercise—walks (20 miles without fatigue), pushes wheelchair, denies sports, regular exercise
   6. Driving—none

F. Sexual History
He has sex only with women, regularly uses condoms for the past 5 years, and understands the need for safe sexual practices.

   E. Health habits
      1. Nutrition
      2. Alcohol (ETOH) use
      3. Smoking
      4. Sleep
      5. Exercise
      6. Driving
   F. Sexual history

REVIEW OF SYSTEMS

The review of systems (ROS) is the format most likely to be included in the acute admitting health history. The ROS (Box 3.16) is a logical "head to toe" overview of what the patient reports about his or her health during the interview. It is not a physical assessment. It can, however, be done at the time of an admitting assessment. Observations made by the nurse or other examiner may lead to what we call "oh, by the way . . ." information. These data may be an ongoing concern of the patient but have been omitted from the verbal interview.

   A. General status
   B. Skin, hair, nails
   C. Eyes
   D. Ears
   E. Nose, sinus
   F. Mouth, throat
   G. Breasts
   H. Respiratory
   I. Cardiovascular
   J. Gastrointestinal
   K. Urinary tract
   L. Genital
   M. Musculoskeletal
   N. Nervous
   O. Endocrine
   P. Hematologic
   Q. Psychological status
   R. OB/GYN

BOX 3.15

"By the Way"

We have found that patients frequently remember pertinent information as you, or they, are walking out the door. We call it "Oh, by the way . . ." data. It is not uncommon for a patient to say, "By the way, I have noticed a funny feeling in my chest when I use the stairs instead of the elevator." If you have ever wondered why you are having difficulty with time management, or have long waiting periods for a doctor's appointment, "oh, by the ways . . ." may be responsible.

There is no simple solution to this problem. Good interviewing techniques and language that helps the patient to recall and report appropriately do help. In the instances when vital information is added in this offhand manner you must be prepared to address the issue and solicit pertinent details.

BOX 3.16

Review of Systems

A. General Status—"feels very healthy."

B. Skin, Hair, Nails—neg. changes in hair and nails, growths, pruritis, color, or rashes.

C. Eyes—alternate dry, irritated and watery, no itching, redness, pain, discharge, burning. Visual acuity good. Family history of cataracts, glaucoma unknown, no diplopia, spots, halos, flashes, temporary blindness.

D. Ears—neg. excess cerumen, discharge, infections, pain. No hearing loss or vertigo.

E. Nose, Sinus—States clear drainage from nose. No epistaxis, sinus discomfort, congestion.

F. Mouth, Throat—Denies any bleeding or sore on gums or tongue. Bilateral second molar extractions to relieve toothache while in jail, otherwise teeth unremarkable. States sore throat when smoking, relieved by cough drops. Neg. hoarseness, frequent URI.

G. Breasts—No lumps, pain, discharge.

H. Respiratory—See HPI. Neg. for asthma, sputum production, wheezing, pleuritic pain.

I. Cardiovascular—No chest pain, palpitations, dyspnea, orthopnea, PND. Peripheral vascular—Neg. claudication, varicosities, phlebitis, edema, color temperature changes.

J. Gastrointestinal—occasional flatulence with milk ingestion, occasional constipation. No eructation, dysphagia, heartburn, indigestion, nausea, vomiting, hematemesis, abdominal pain, diarrhea. BMs —1/day, brown, formed, denies melena, BRBPR.

K. Urinary Tract—Neg. for dysuria, nocturia, pyuria, frequency, urgency, change in stream, hesitancy, incontinence, stones.

L. Genital—See HPI. No urethral discharge, penile or scrotal lesions or swelling, testicular pain or swelling, impotence. Does not do testicular self-exam.

M. Musculoskeletal—see PHH; denies swelling, fractures, sprains, deformities.

N. Nervous—Neg. syncope, seizures, vertigo, speech difficulties, gait problems, ataxia, tremor, muscle weakness, tingling, numbness, headache.

O. Endocrine—No tremor, heat or cold intolerance, change in voice, glove or shoe size, polydipsia, polyuria, polyphagia.

P. Hematologic—No spontaneous bleeding or bruising, easy bruising.

Q. Psychological Status—See HPI. Hands sweat and feet get cold when anxious. Neg. for mood swings, preoccupations, apathy, memory disturbance, nervousness, difficulty concentrating, suicidal ideation.

R. OB/GYN—Not applicable.

ORDER AND ORGANIZATION

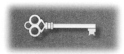

When you perform a physical assessment related to a complaint or patient status change, how do you know that your assessment is complete? This is especially an issue if the evaluation reveals no obvious physical change or "cause." When charting, how do you decide what information is relevant to include in the patient's record? If you can devise a system that allows you to proceed with a sense of organization, a sense of order, the outcome will be more consistent assessments and inclusive documentation. Thinking in order leads to charting in order. Efficiency and accuracy within your practice become easier to achieve.

Most patients have heads and most patients have toes. The inherent and instructional order of the CHH and PE is to document assessment data in a "head to toe" format. This "head to toe" process of interview and assessment is a key to your learning how to chart. This logical order will help you develop information-gathering skills. Proficiency will be gained through repetition. You will notice that charting becomes easier and more fluid as you practice with this consistent and methodical format.

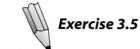

Exercise 3.5

Organize each group of "positive" symptoms in a "head to toe" order. An actual ROS will consist of both positives and negatives that you may need to synopsize for report. Don't worry about prioritizing at this time. You are only working to develop a systematic method of organizing data. Later you will integrate organization with prioritization and nursing process.

1. Patient A
   Feels "tired," headaches q 2–3 days, numbness and tingling both feet, heartburn p̄ dinner, frequent urination.

2. Patient B
   Swollen ankles, rash on buttocks, morning and evening cough, nightly leg cramps.

3. Patient C
   Heavy menstrual flow, double vision, low back pain, fatigue

4. Patient D
   Difficulty breathing, no appetite, frequent cold sores on lips and tongue, painful varicose veins, dizziness on standing

5. Patient E
   Abdominal cramping p̄ meals, tinnitus q AM × 30 min, rash L axilla, poor appetite.

PROBLEM LIST

The CHH concludes with a problem list. It typically includes all major health issues beginning with health maintenance. Problems are listed in descending order from current and active to earlier resolved and ongoing health problems (Box 3.17). Health maintenance issues are always considered ongoing and are properly addressed by qualified health care professionals who have patient contact.

Date	Problem	Onset	Resolved
	1. Health maintenance		

BOX 3.17

Problem List

Date Recorded	Established Problem	Onset	Resolved
10/93	1. Health Maintenance		
10/93	2. Smoking	1988	
10/93	3. Situational Life Stress	1993	
10/93	4. + PPD, possible active TB	1993	

Status Post

1. HBV—1988

STATUS POST

The "status post" lists past health problems that have been resolved and are not considered to affect current care. An example might be a past fracture or surgery with no sequelae. Learn the difference between "status post" and "concurrent" problems. "Status post" means that a problem has been resolved.

VERBAL REPORT/SUMMARY

The verbal report (Box 3.18) is a short, one minute or less, review of the patient's history. It may include the facts from a physical exam if one has been

---

BOX 3.18

Verbal Report

33 y/o Hispanic single unemployed male referred with positive PPD, night sweats times 5 months, decreased appetite with 15 pound wt. loss, fever. Negative for fatigue, cough, sputum production, hemoptysis, dyspnea, chest pain, allergies. Active problems include cocaine abuse, cigarette use (4 pack years), situational life stress. PHH positive for HBV 1988, gonorrhea 1988. FH, OH noncontributory. P/SH significant for ETOH intake, anxiety, past high risk behavior, lack of financial, medical support

ROS notable for smoking-related sore throat, constipation. Patient appears healthy, without acute symptoms, T 37°C, P 72, BP lying 120/70, R 16. No significant findings on physical exam.

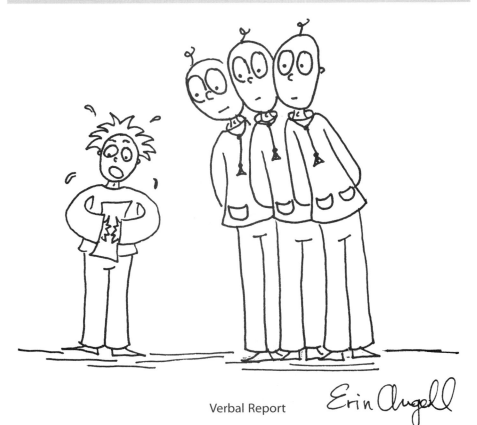

Verbal Report

Erin Angell

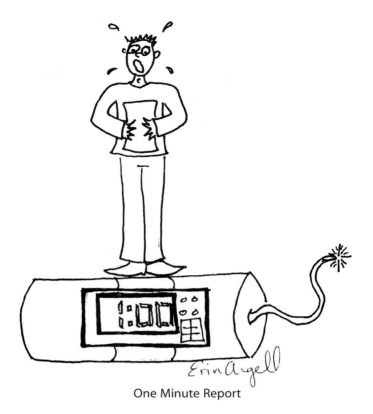

One Minute Report

BOX 3.19

Speaking Confidently

Fear of public speaking and hesitant speech patterns can impede the delivery of a verbal report. Other speech habits that may lead to poor verbal reporting are frequent use of "uh" and "um," or reliance on slang, such as "you know" or "whatchamacallit." Learning to deliver, or "give" a professional sounding report to other team members is not handed to you with your uniform or diploma. It is a learned and acquired skill.

The lack of clear instruction in language and delivery technique is one of the least recognized, yet most important, impediments to learning to give a verbal report. Time constraints on nursing programs coupled with increasing didactic content leaves little time for the instructor to cover details of charting and report.

Another problem is the "correction" method of teaching, in which you chart or give report and are then corrected. For many of us, this type of learning can lead to withdrawing from opportunities for experiences to document or deliver report. There is potential to create even greater difficulties with hesitance or speech patterns.

A solution to these problems is to practice written and verbal documentation using your organized format. Write notes for the case studies you read in your texts and do a verbal report in a recorder or in front of a classmate. Strengthen your organizational format by repetition and practice until you gain confidence. With confidence comes proficiency. Determining your organizational style allows you to put the data you have gathered into familiar order. Knowing your data, knowing how you always organize it will improve your charting skills and will give you increased confidence with verbal report.

done. This is an area in which verbal language and nursing process are put together to communicate coherently. You are once again learning to practice with a format familiar to other caregivers.

The summary is the written counterpart to the verbal report, found at the end of the Complete Health History (Box 3.20). It is a snapshot, a brief overview, which presents the pertinent details about the patient.

Exercise 3.6

You are a nurse in a clinic and are required to present a brief description of each patient to the primary care provider before they meet the patient. Using data from the word list, fill in the information in parentheses to complete the patient summary. You can use these summaries to practice verbal report!

(Name), profile, pt. of (provider) presented with/current complaint, describe complaint, vital signs/pertinent lab values, supporting factors from ROS, contributing factors, interventions, outcomes

1. Patient A
   T 102°F
   difficulty swallowing
   patient of Dr. M
   + quick strep

   Ms. B., 22 y/o, w, F, _____, presents with sore throat, _____, VS_____, 110/80, 72, 16, _____, swollen tonsils, irritable, 6 y/o child status post strep throat, antiseptic gargle bid, no relief of pain.

2. Patient B
   c/o diarrhea
   OTC antacid no relief
   M (male)
   36 y/o

   Mr. D., _____, NA (Native American), _____, pt of Dr. M, _____, nausea and vomiting × 36 hrs c̄ moderate LLQ "cramps," T 100°F, 145/78, 88, 14, − diet Δ or food allergies, _____.

3. Patient C
   sexually active
   F
   severe suprapubic
   22, shallow

   Ms. C, 18 y/o, _____, admitted from ER (Emergency Room), _____, abdominal pain, 8/10, no rebound, T 99°F, 130/88, 94, _____, LNMP (last normal menstrual period) mid-June, _____, + pregnancy, neg. precautions/birth control

4. Patient D
   c/o relentless
   75 y/o
   no relief
   c̄ restlessness

   Ms. D, _____, CCU pt. of Dr. G, ESRF (end stage renal failure), _____, severe urticaria (itching), _____, medicated at 0300, _____, request new orders from MD.

5. Patient E
   O₂ at 2 liters
   126/88

BOX 3.20

Complete Health History

Informant

Patient Profile

Objective description of patient, purpose for seeking medical care, who they are

Chief Complaint

Quote direct from patient perspective

History of Present Illness

Location, radiation, quality, quantity, timing, setting, aggravating/relieving factors, associated manifestations, meaning to patient

Concurrent Health Problems

Chronological list of ongoing heath issues not necessarily related to current problem

Past Health History

A. Childhood
  1. Communicable diseases
  2. Illness/accidents/injuries
  3. Surgery
B. Adulthood
  1. Illness
    a. Medical
    b. Occupational/litigation
  2. Surgery
  3. Accidents/injuries
  4. Psychiatric
  5. Allergies
  6. Medications
    a. Rx
    b. OTC
  7. Immunizations
  8. Screening/prevention
    a. PPD
    b. Mammography
    c. Other
  9. Dental
  10. Eye
  11. Additional risk factors
    a. Travel
    b. Transfusions
    c. Exposures
    d. Other

Family History

Occupational/Environmental History

Personal/Social History

A. Family/cultural influences
B. Education
C. Marital/relationship history
D. Current life situation
E. Health habits
  1. Nutrition
  2. Alcohol (ETOH) use
  3. Smoking
  4. Sleep
  5. Exercise
  6. Driving
F. Sexual history

Review of Systems

A. General status
B. Skin, hair, nails
C. Eyes
D. Ears
E. Nose, sinus
F. Mouth, throat
G. Breasts
H. Respiratory
I. Cardiovascular
J. Gastrointestinal
K. Urinary tract
L. Genital
M. Musculoskeletal
N. Nervous
O. Endocrine
P. Hematologic
Q. Psychological status
R. OB/GYN

Problem List

Date	Problem	Onset	Resolved
	1. Health maintenance		

Status Post

Summary

airway patent
ER admit post MVA (motor vehicle accident)
lips dusky

Mr. E, 26 y/o, _____, multiple fractures, c/o difficulty breathing, _____,
shallow breath sounds bilateral R 26, _____, restlessness, P 96, T 98°F,
_____, head elevated to 30° c̄ no relief, _____, ER physician notified.

Make copies of the CHH (Box 3.20) to use for your patient interview. Or create a form that meets your clinical needs. Sample forms are included at the end of the chapter.

Answer Guide

Exercise 3.1

1. collateral
   Common: corroborating, supporting, indirect
   Technical: subsidiary to primary, as with arteries

2. coping
   Common: top of wall
   Technical: ability to face problem and resolve it

3. digit
   Common: number
   Technical: finger or toe

4. flush
   Common: to flow copiously; to blush or turn red; poker hand with cards all in the same suit; hunting term for exposing game birds; to wash out a toilet with copious amounts of water
   Technical: to irrigate or wash out with large amounts of water

5. lacerate
   Common: rip; tear
   Technical: tear tissue; wound with jagged edge

6. lacrimation
   Common: secretion of tears
   Technical: tears

7. lactate
   Common: to secrete milk
   Technical: a product of lactic acid; to produce milk

8. lead
   Common: to guide or direct; to be at head; dull gray metal
   Technical: connection for electrical conduction usually between a patient and measuring device

9. macerate
   Common: to soak in liquid to soften and separate into components
   Technical: to soften or make thin

10. maintain
    Common: to continue; to keep in good condition
    Technical: to comply with good health practice

11. nonresponsive
    Common: to not reply, not react
    Technical: no reaction, physical or mental, to applied stimulus

12. patent
    Common: government document that ensures inventor's rights; the obvious
    Technical: opened, not plugged

13. phalanx
    Common: A tightly grouped formation
    Technical: singular for long bones of fingers

14. piggyback
    Common: position in which one person carries another on shoulders; truck trailer carried on the flat car of train
    Technical: to deliver a bag of IV solution by injecting into existing IV tubing

15. run
    Common: to move rapidly on foot; to compete for an elected office; to drive or steer
    Technical: to deliver fluids or medications through IV

16. stool
    Common: seat with no back or arms; footrest
    Technical: fecal material

17. titrate
    Common: determine solution concentration
    Technical: deliver solution in a specific concentration over a defined time period

18. transpose
    Common: to change or reverse the order of
    Technical: to replace existing IV fluid bag with a new or different bag; to change placement of organs or tissue

19. turn
    Common: move or cause to move
    Technical: change patient position on a regular schedule

20. vapors
    Common: gaseous state of a normally liquid or solid matter; old-fashioned term for feeling poorly
    Technical: inhaled medication

21. void
    Common: empty; unoccupied
    Technical: to urinate or defecate

22. pattern
    Common: design or model; routine way of doing things
    Technical: recognizable model; repetitive behavior trait

Exercise 3.2

1. Mr. X, 55 y/o, black, M, married, self employed Navy retiree, admitted for L inguinal hernia.

2. Mrs. X, 80 y/o, white, F, widow (3 months, 5 children, pt. of Dr. ABC, admitted for R heart failure.

3. X. Y., 17 y/o, Asian, M, intact family, 1 sister, admitted for testicular tumor, R.

4. Ms. Y, 35 y/o, white, F, married, 2 children, admitted for L breast mass.
   (May be Jewish, but there is no clear statement here.)

5. Y. Z., 5 months, F, Chinese, admitted for respiratory dysfunction, accompanied by sister and aunt who is interpreting. Parents working.
   (This history would show the sister or aunt as narrator. Family information, in this case, is important in diagnosing and planning care for this infant.)

Exercise 3.3

1. b, 2. b, 3. b, 4. b, 5. a

Exercise 3.4

1. CAD (coronary artery disease)
2. HTN (hypertension)
3. CVD (cardiovascular disease)
4. DM (diabetes mellitus)
5. TB (tuberculosis)
6. CA (cancer)
7. HA (headache)

Exercise 3.5

1. Feels "tired," headaches q 2–3 days, heartburn $\bar{p}$ dinner, frequent urination, numbness and tingling in both feet.
2. Rash on buttocks, morning and evening cough, swollen ankles, nightly leg cramps
3. Fatigue, double vision, "hot flashes," low back pain, heavy menstrual flow
4. No appetite, frequent cold sores on lips and tongue, painful varicose veins, dizziness on standing
5. Poor appetite, rash L axilla, tinnitus q AM × 30 min, abdominal cramping $\bar{p}$ meals

Exercise 3.6

1. Patient A
   patient of Dr. M
   difficulty swallowing
   102°F
   + quick strep
2. Patient B
   36 y/o
   m (male)
   diarrhea
   OTC antacid no relief
3. Patient C
   F
   22, shallow
   severe suprapubic
   sexually active
4. Patient D
   75 y/o
   c/o relentless
   $\bar{c}$ restlessness
   no relief
5. Patient E
   ER admit post MVA (motor vehicle accident)
   airway patent
   lips dusky
   O_2 at 2 liters
   126/88

Sample chart 1.

HEALTH ASSESSMENT

Name: _____

Date: _____

Time: _____

Patient Profile

Association with health care facility:

Age:____   Sex:____   Race:____

Marital Status:_____   Employment Status:_____

Diagnoses / Other:

_____

_____

Chief Complaint:

_____
_____
_____
_____
_____
_____
_____

Present Illness:

Health Status	**Supporting Data**
Location/Radiation:	ROS:
Quality:	PH:
Intensity:	FH:
Duration/Frequency:	P/SH:

Functional Status:

Psychological Impact:

Patient's Theory:

Sample chart 2.

NAME: _____

Date: _____

<u>CHIEF COMPLAINT</u>: Pt is a _____ yr. old _____ pt. of

Character:

Location:

Onset:

Duration:

Worse:

Relief:

<u>REVIEW OF SYSTEMS</u>

<u>Positive</u>   <u>Negative</u>

PAST MEDICAL HISTORY

<u>Positive</u>   <u>Negative</u>

Family History:

Medications:

Allergies:

Smoke:

Alcohol:

Personal/Social History:

PHYSICAL EXAM

ASSESSMENT

PLANS

Sample chart 3.

HEALTH ASSESSMENT

Past Medical History
General State of Health_____
Childhood Illnesses_____
Immunizations:

tetanus_____	German measles_____
pertussis_____	mumps_____
diptheria_____	flu_____
polio_____	pneumonia_____
measles_____	

Major Adult Illnesses_____
Operations_____
Injuries_____
Other Hospitilizations_____
Obstetrical History_____
Current Medications, Home remedies etc_____
Coffee, Alcohol, Tobacco, other drugs_____
Allergies, Drug Sensitivities_____

Family and Genetic History
Age & Health or Cause of Death

Mother_____	Spouse_____
Father_____	Children_____
Siblings_____	Grandparents_____

Occurrence of Chronic Health Conditions in Immediate Family Members

	cancer_____
diabetes_____	arthritis_____
tuberculosis_____	anemia_____
heart disease_____	headaches_____
high blood pressure_____	nervous disorders_____
stroke_____	mental illness_____
renal disease_____	like symptoms_____

Psychosocial History

Date of Birth	Home situation
Places of Residence	Significant Others / Support System
Educational History	Religious and Cultural Beliefs
Significant Experiences:	Job History
(childhood/adolescence)	Travel and Military History
Marital History	Use of Leisure Time
Values / Attitudes Regarding Sexuality	Financial Status
Feelings about self as:	Sources of Satisfaction and Distress
Masculine / Feminine	Typical Day
Current Lifestyle	

CHAPTER 4

Beginning Well

WORD LIST

alter	incontinent	needleless
atraumatic	intolerance	potential
calf	invasive	status
compress	main	trauma
deficit	met	tube
impaired	morbid	valve
implant	moribund	obtunded

 Exercise 4.1

Each item in the word list has both common and technical meanings. Match each word with its corresponding set of definitions and compare the intent or usage of the terms as both common and technical words.

1. _____
   Common: change; tailor; castrate or spay
   Technical: change

2. _____
   Common: no trauma
   Technical: without trauma

3. _____
   Common: baby, young cow
   Technical: muscular area of the lower portion of the leg

4. _____
   Common: condense
   Technical: pads or gauze applied for pressure, heat, or cold

5. _____
   Common: shortfall of money; inadequate
   Technical: insufficient; that which is being consumed faster than replaced

6. _____
   Common: to set firmly; instill
   Technical: graft; insert in tissue; put in surgically

7. _____
   Common: not controlled; unable to be restrained
   Technical: unable to control excretory functions

8. _____
   Common: denoting an the act of violating; tending to overrun harmfully
   Technical: denoting a puncture, incision, or penetration of the body; relating to the spread of neoplasm to adjoining tissue

9. _____
   Common: most important; large pipe or conduit
   Technical: primary source, such as coronary arteries

10. _____
    Common: past tense of the word *meet*
    Technical: shortened form of the word *metastasis* (spread or implant of neoplasm to other tissue)

11. _____
    Common: gruesome, grisly; unwholesome preoccupation
    Technical: related to disease; deviant

12. _____
    Common: near death
    Technical: dying; death imminent

13. _____
    Common: no needle
    Technical: any system which has been modified to eliminate needle use

14. _____
    Common: latent; expected capacity for development
    Technical: possible but not real; action which may take place under proscribed conditions

15. _____
    Common: legal definition of state of person or thing; high social regard
    Technical: condition; assessment of patient state

16. _____
    Common: wound
    Technical: wound or shock; injury accidental or purposefully inflicted

17. _____
    Common: pipe; hollow cylinder
    Technical: canal; hollow organ; or any pipe through which oxygen, medication, or food is given, or fluid drained from body orifice

18. _____
    Common: structure which regulates the flow of gas or liquid
    Technical: membrane of canal or hollow organ that prevents reflux of fluid

19. _____
    Common: diminished; harmed
    Technical: weakened; damaged; deteriorated

20. _____
    Common: unbearable nature; bigotry
    Technical: inability to handle substance or inability to endure

21. _____
    Common: oblivious to external stimuli
    Technical: reduced level of consciousness due to analgesia, or use of drugs or alcohol

USING LANGUAGE IN YOUR CLINICAL PRACTICE

Clinical practice exercises in this chapter should be concurrent with clinical practicum in your nursing program. You are now prepared to conduct an introductory patient interview, take vital signs, and provide assistance with activities of daily living (ADLs). The documentation exercises in this chapter might also be practiced as part of your skills lab. Case studies begin in this chapter to reinforce language skills necessary for recording nursing tasks.

The case study exercises focus on acute care, clinic, and skilled nursing settings. Your task in working with the case studies is to organize patient data, practice charting, and prepare a verbal report. The case study drills help you develop the language skills necessary for recording nursing tasks.

The broad focus of this case study information addresses the needs of the beginning student as well as those of the nurse experienced in basic patient care. The case studies are exercises in documentation and not intended to be a test of your theoretical knowledge. In the initial cases, key information is highlighted. As you become familiar with the case study process, key information will not be highlighted. Preliminary case studies are intentionally designed to limit your application of critical thinking skills into language, vocabulary, and organization of key information.

All nurses need to understand the consequences of including or excluding proper descriptive data in the patient chart. Nursing education focuses on bedside interventions related to your foundation in pathophysiology and technical procedures. Your knowledge base is dependent on information that you learn in theory-based classes, and applied to data collected from your coworkers, the patient's chart, and especially from interviewing and assessing the patient. However, the most thorough understanding of your patient is rendered useless if you are unable to characterize the information in a way that best describes the patient's response to his or her illness. For instance, shortness of breath (SOB) can be an indicator of a disease process as well as an expected physiologic response to certain strenuous activity.

You have learned that by developing and using a routine format you can avoid errors of omission and you can improve your prioritization skills. Once you have a format to follow you also have a plan for asking questions. Critical

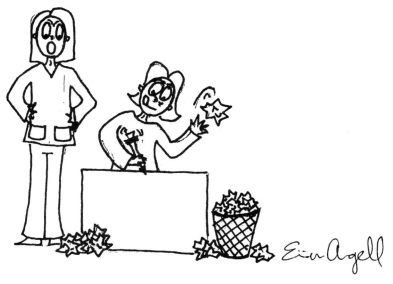

"Are you done yet?"

thinking enables you to discern what data to collect. If it were necessary to quote the patient interview exactly it would be more expedient to audiotape the conversation. Practice and repetition will reinforce your ability to record in precise language that which is essential. By prioritizing collected data and using professional judgment regarding what should be documented in the patient's chart, you will learn to chart exactly what is necessary.

You may begin your clinical documentation practice by recording vital signs. Your initial observations will also involve observing the patient in his or her room. This is your opportunity to visually assess and determine personal patient data remarkable for documentation. Temperature, blood pressure, pulse, and respiration are measurable, objective findings. Vital signs need no further description as long as they remain within normal or expected range. If they are found to be abnormal or "deviant," then additional information may be necessary. You may need to describe the quality or nature of these unexpected parameters while recording data that support your assessment findings.

For example, abnormal pulse findings can be detected by palpation or assessed through cardiac auscultation. The nursing note should reflect the origin of the finding by stating the pulse's point of origin, i.e., apical or radial. Your note should also include the nature of the sound and character of the heartbeat. If the findings are consistent with previous assessment or present no change in the patient's status, then no further documentation is warranted. If the findings are new or different, then documentation must include a plan of action with expected outcome. Follow-up notes record the interventions and the actual outcome. To complete the documentation picture, it is necessary to record nursing assessment, plan, actions, and evaluation.

Imagine you are a detective looking for patient clues, which we will call signs and symptoms. As a nurse investigator, you are seeking the information that allows you to plan patient care. Your investigation may lead you to the solution of the problem or it will help you to uncover further, important clues relevant to the patient's condition. Here is a sample of questions you might use to uncover patient clues.

What is the admitting problem?

What nursing interventions are applicable?

What changes are observed in patient status?

What caused the change?

Is the change in response to treatment or intervention?

How did the patient respond to the change?

What interventions need to be changed in response to the patient's condition?

What outcome is your most desirable nursing diagnosis?

What is your plan to evaluate your interventions?

Were your nursing interventions effective?

NURSING DIAGNOSIS

Nursing diagnoses are written with standardized language and in a format that provides a universal model for understanding what nurses do. It is the first step in teaching nurses to use a common language. You must be clear in your comprehension of the words used by the North American Nursing Diagnosis Association (NANDA) to understand each nursing diagnosis.

The NANDA model focuses on nursing diagnoses (ND). ND are selected based upon a patient's nursing needs, as determined by the nurse. As you are learning the language and application of NANDA, you will note the repetitive use of actionable words. Do you recognize these NANDA action words?

deficit: inadequate; insufficient

altered: changed

impaired: diminished in value or usefulness

risk for: possibility of harm or damage

intolerance: inability to bear; incompatibility with

ineffective: not working as anticipated; not useful

less than/more than body requirements: incompatible with individual physical needs

effective: that which results in positive outcome

potential for: possibility of occurrence; likely to be a result of

You need to know the meaning of these terms as they relate to nursing. You must conceptually understand their intent. Some of the words have subtle differences between meaning and intent. Match the terms below in Exercise 4.2 with their action-based meaning.

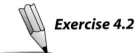

Exercise 4.2

deficit

potential for

effective

less than/more than body requirements

ineffective

intolerance

risk for

altered

impaired

1. inadequate; insufficient
2. changed
3. diminished in value or usefulness
4. possibility of harm or damage
5. unable to bear; incompatible with
6. not working as anticipated; not useful
7. incompatible with individual physical needs
8. that which results in positive outcome
9. possibility of occurrence; likely to be a result of

SYNTAX

Syntax is the way in which words are put together. It is the format of a sentence. Nursing documentation does not necessarily follow the rules of grammatical syntax for a sentence, phrase, or clause. The syntax of your charted note will reflect the nature and importance of the information you are sharing. The structure of your written or verbal report is designed to communicate with health care professionals working toward a common goal.

While learning the structure of NANDA, you will also learn to recognize the syntax chosen for designating a specific nursing diagnosis (ND). The first word of each ND is the identified problem or potential problem. This problem is followed by words that imply nursing actions or potential nursing actions applicable to the particular problem.

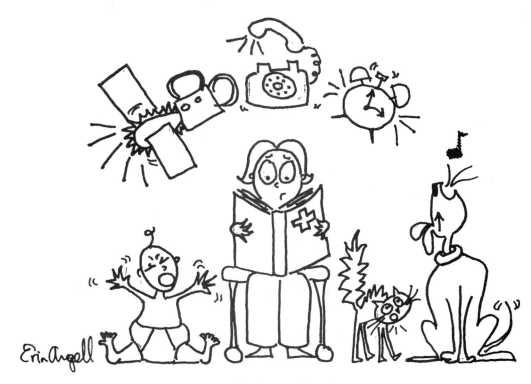

Coping, ineffective

In order to understand a ND you need knowledge relative to the character-ized pathology. As an example, consider the phrase "coping, individual, ineffec-tive." To a nontechnical reader these are three disparate words expressing no co-hesive idea or thought; to health care professionals, it means much more. As nurses, we know that "coping" refers to the state of managing a stressful event. We understand that the term "individual" isolates the problem to one person or patient rather than to a group of people. The third word, "ineffective," declares that the coping style for this patient is considered by the nursing staff to be "not working" in a safe or healthy way.

NANDA is thus more than groups of words arranged in a bizarre syntax. It is a roadmap that can guide the nurse to apply the proper skills for patient prob-lem resolution. Specific interventions are considered appropriate relative to how the patient is managing his or her stress. If you understand how NANDA orga-nizes technical words and associate those words with the actions they imply, you can more consistently apply the nursing process.

SYNTAX, NURSING NOTES

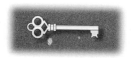

There are no formal rules of syntax common in nursing at the present time. As you develop your skills and learn an organized format you will also be deter-mining rules to govern your own thought processes. In effect you will be devel-oping a style for organizing thought, which will be mirrored in the syntax of your charted data.

This workbook uses the CHH and head-to-toe order for documentation. It has defined specific tenets of effective charting: *prioritization, organization, rele-vancy, brevity, accuracy, and efficiency.* Syntax becomes the tool you use to put it all together. Syntax is about choosing and expressing words with the goal of documenting collected information clearly. You are working to refine these learned tools in order to establish effective and organized professional practice standards. These will contribute to enhanced time management skills.

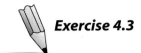 **Exercise 4.3**

Examine the syntax of the following NANDA entries. Match them with the appropriate corresponding data set.

Airway, ineffective

Gas exchange, impaired

Protection, altered

Nutrition, less than body requirements

Infection, risk for

1. Pt. A, 88 y/o, M, esophageal stricture, persistent vomiting at meals, 20 lb. wt. loss × 3 weeks.
2. Pt. B, 17 mo., F, pneumonia, LLL [left lower lobe], dusky, irritable.
3. Pt. C, 5 y/o, severe asthma, R 30, shallow
4. Pt. D, 72 y/o, F, post-op, ORIF rt. hip fx [fracture], general anesthesia
5. Pt. E, 35 y/o, M, third degree chemical burn 40% back and neck

INTRODUCING DESCRIPTOR WORDS

You are now familiar with the tools used to organize your assessment and to keep the narration clear and concise. You are ready to use your judgment in modifying your assessment to accurately reflect patient status.

In written English, modifiers are adjectives, adverbs, and phrases which complete a descriptive picture. In nursing, modifiers used in addition to the basic facts are called descriptors or symptom descriptors. Symptom descriptors are used judiciously in progress notes in order to present a complete picture of patient status. Chapter 2 discussed vague or incomplete charting. Chapter 8 will detail important medical and legal tenets of documentation. You are now learning to modify the most fundamental data for definition and clarification. The

---

BOX 4.1

Quantification: Measuring a Response

We are introducing the concept of quantifying, or measuring, a patient's response. While chapters 5 and 6 will go into great detail, it is necessary for you to understand the word *quantify* in regard to using modifiers in your note. This will help you avoid vague incomprehensible charting.

Since "pain" is a symptom that you will be exposed to from your first clinical it can be used as a useful example. "Pain" usually refers to an actual physical or mental sensation of discomfort. Informally it alludes to the actual meaning by inferring that something that is a pain is difficult or a nuisance. Consequently you must describe or "quantify" the word *pain* in your note to give it the precise meaning you intend.

medical record is no place for inadequate or inaccurate documentation. Descriptors are a means to better quantify your professional judgment and findings.

For instance, a notation which reads "c/o pain" requires descriptive words to modify or explain exactly what the note means. "Pain" by itself is a word that implies a need for nursing intervention. This note, however, does not tell you anything about the location, severity, onset, duration, or quality of the symptom the patient calls "pain." It does not tell you what relieves it or what makes it worse. Using a note that reads "c/o pain" and leaving it unmodified is like trying to make a cake with only one ingredient. It cannot work.

Specific and objective descriptors provide you with the "ingredients" to complete your note. There are no written rules to guide your choice and use of descriptors. You will be relying on your judgment and experience to determine which descriptors are necessary and objective. Guidelines are provided in Chapter 2 with regard to your interviewing skills. A more detailed guide for symptom descriptor use will be presented in Chapter 6.

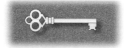

The etiology of the symptom is clarified when you include descriptors. Consider the example: "c/o pain." If you add a descriptor to specify the location of the pain, your note becomes: "c/o chest pain." You may further state: "c/o midsternal chest pain." Details make the difference. You might modify further: "c/o midsternal chest pain radiating to jaw, L shoulder, and arm."

You now have a very vivid description, which should initiate specific and rapid interventions. In this example, each added modifier is necessary and succinct. The syntax of the statement "positions" the modifiers so that anyone reading the note can visualize the pain pattern. There are no extraneous words and no confusion. Your choice of descriptors influences the nature and urgency of your patient's care.

Reread the example. Does the patient always tell the nurse that he or she was experiencing pain? Or do the fine points of the patient's complaint come with investigation? The factual information in the completed note may develop after the patient states "I'm fine, but am a little uncomfortable." *Your* attention to detail makes a difference.

SIMPLE CHARTING: A BEGINNING

You are ready to begin applying your language and syntax skills to charting your nursing interventions. You will be charting in the patient's progress notes, while still in the process of learning didactic content in nursing theory. It might be easier to approach this learning task as you do hand skills, that is, by gradually building skills on a foundation of current knowledge.

Hand skills are gradually introduced into the lab curriculum. Each new skill you learn may "borrow" techniques learned from earlier skills. For instance, you learn about clean and sterile technique in one of your initial skills classes and then apply this information to subsequent skills such as irrigation, dressing changes, or injections.

Similarly, you will begin charting in a progressive and simple manner. As your assessment skills expand you become comfortable with your mastery of those skills. Your charting will also reflect your increased level of expertise. In the meantime, practice applying the language and syntax skills as you develop new skills.'

Case Study 4.1a

Your patient is a 33-year-old man who was admitted the previous evening through the emergency room. He was diagnosed with appendicitis and was taken to surgery for an appendectomy. He is now one day postoperative on the medical-surgical unit.

Your clinical objective for the day is to take vital signs and to provide morning (AM) care. You are encouraged to practice your CHH interviewing skills as you assist the patient with bathing, oral hygiene, and meals. This is your first clinical experience that involves patient care, and you realize that your knowledge base is limited. Your clinical instructor is available on the unit for assistance and support.

Your personal goals for the day's clinical:

- to appear professional
- to complete the "hands on" tasks
- to be prepared to report to the patient's primary nurse
- to complete your charting in time for your clinical post-conference

Case Study 4.1b

Your patient is receptive to having you as part of the team and cooperates with no complaint. When you ask your patient how he feels, you learn that he is worried about his employer being notified about his absence from work. He has been working on a project that was scheduled for completion in two weeks' time. He then states that he is having "belly" pain and points to his incision site. He also complains of "occasional" feelings of nausea, with no urge to vomit. You make sure that the patient is safe in his bed with an emesis basin close by. The bed is in its lowered position with side rails up. You seek help from your instructor.

You and your clinical instructor find the staff nurse assigned to your patient and you report your findings. You are ready to chart your activities. You begin by noting the patient's complaint and all interventions in the written progress notes. The facility has a patient checklist for recording daily care activities (remember ADLs). You will also need to write a note documenting the outcome of your intervention or action.

You use the checklist to initial the tasks that you performed or assisted the patient to accomplish. These may include vital signs and ADLs such as meals consumed, voiding and bowel movements, and safety precautions. You are now faced with the task of charting additional select information in the written progress notes. What to do? Where to start?

SIMPLE CHARTING: A MIDDLE

Think of your format! Is it necessary to write a patient profile? Probably not! Format the priority information in your mind and practice by writing it out on scratch paper.

Here is what you remember about your preliminary patient visit:

Time of patient contact: 1000

Presenting complaint: R abdominal pain or pain RLQ

Associated factors: nausea, no vomiting (pertinent negative) (if both nausea and vomiting are problems, N & V can be used)

Interventions: emesis basin, side rails up, bed lowered, staff notified

Outcome of interventions: staff nurse to assess patient for c/o pain and nausea

You make an entry into the patient record. Your note now reads: "1000: c/o pain RLQ, +nausea, −vomiting, emesis basin, [record safety precautions if not on checklist], staff consulted and responding."

Note the syntax of the note. Single words express complete thoughts. With minimal rhetoric you have recorded all necessary information. As you proceed in school, your nursing skills will also progress. You will be assessing a patient's pain, the surgical dressings, nutritional and hydration status, as well as performing nursing interventions. You will also learn to record the effectiveness of any intervention. As a beginning nurse your written note usually includes known patient data, even if the data are not clinically complete. In order for the note to be clinically complete patient symptoms would need to be modified using select, descriptive words.

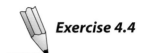 **Exercise 4.4**

Read the following chart entries. The highlighted entries belong to one of the following categories:

Complaint (C)

Associated Symptoms (A)

Intervention (I)

Outcome (O)

Example: 1100: c/o HA pain (C), N & V (A), staff consulted (I) & responding (O).

1. 0800: c/o light sensitivity OU ____, lights dimmed ____, curtain drawn ____, staff consulted ____.
2. 2100: c/o pain IV site L wrist ____, redness ____, swelling ____, cool to touch ____, IV d'c'd ____, warm compress applied ____.
3. 2200: ↓ pain ____, redness ____, swelling ____, L wrist, d'c warm compress ____.
4. 0630: c/o itching & burning ____, RLQ, dressing dry & intact, staff consulted ____ & responding ____.
5. 0730: dressing (drsg) Δ ____, incision red ____, warm ____, thick, yellow drainage ____, T 101°F ____, MD notified ____.

SIMPLE CHARTING: AN END

Words that describe a patient's symptom, or descriptors, will be thoroughly explained in Chapter 6. Reread the charted note above. The "incision site" for an appendectomy is located in the right lower quadrant of the abdomen (Figure 4.1). The note reads only "RLQ." This descriptor stands alone, that is, by itself it conveys information regarding the location of the pain. Further assessment will determine other data to include about the pain.

Figure 4.1

RUQ	**LUQ**
RLQ	**LLQ**

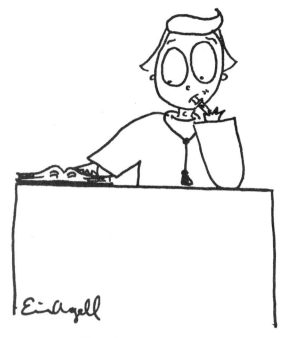

How do you say. . . .

What about the anxiety the patient expressed earlier regarding his work responsibilities? You should read the hospital admission note and the admitting HH (health history). If it is noted, check to see if this problem is being addressed in the nursing diagnoses. You may be responsible for adding a nursing diagnosis and amending the care plan or noting the ND on the clinical pathway. Your instructor and staff will help you to chart this information in the appropriate place so that it will be recognized and addressed before anxiety negatively affects the patient's progress.

BOX 4.2

Nursing Care Plans or Critical Pathways

Many facilities are transitioning from the use of nursing care plans (NCP) to that of clinical pathways (CP). Some have incorporated the NCP into the pathway as the guide for achieving the clinical goals. Others use both as integral but separate means to achieve appropriate patient care.

Once you have learned nursing process, it should be clear that your standard of practice will be defined by your ability to deliver care safely and appropriately regardless of the standardized written plan of action. As you are learning, patients will deviate from the path or respond unexpectedly to an intervention on the care plan. Nurses then reassess their goals to accommodate the individual patient's response to care.

In order to accomplish the reassessment of nursing interventions and adapting care to meet a patient's needs, you will refer to previous nursing notes. The notes which should clearly document the problem, intervention, desired outcome, and actual outcome are the source of information for you to *evaluate* what occurred and create a new plan.

Your key to planning is the historical documentation of patient intervention and outcomes. This is a fluid process that is based on the expectations of how an intervention will succeed in a desired outcome. We standardize in plans or pathways what usually works for most patients considering a given set of circumstances. The individual patient's response to the interventions are the clues, or data set, that allow us to reassess and compare the actual outcome to the expected results. Without good data we are less likely to be able to problem solve for the patient in a timely and effective manner.

Case Study 4.2

Read the case study. Choose the *best* syntax for presenting the information in the multiple choice section.

You have been assigned Patient A, a 59 y/o black woman who was brought to the ER by her family who found her unconscious in the bathroom. She demonstrated left-sided weakness, slight paralysis, and slurred speech and is being "worked up" for CVA. She needs assistance with ADLs and seems frustrated when she speaks. She has lived alone for the past five years and her family says she is very "independent." Her vital signs are WNL with the exception of her blood pressure, which is 150/88. She takes no medicine at home, is postmenopausal, and has worked for the county for 22 years.

After her bath she complains of a "splitting" headache. You turn down the lights and take her blood pressure, which is 180/100. After raising the side rails you look for your instructor or the staff nurse to report.

Choose the best phrasing of the following data:

1. Patient A, _____
   a. black woman, age 59
   b. F, 59 y/o, black
   c. 59 y/o, black, F

2. Found unconscious by family and brought to ER, possible CVA
   a. admitted to ER unconscious with CVA
   b. ER unconscious admit poss. CVA
   c. ER admit, unconscious, r/o [rule out] CVA

3. Left-sided weakness and slurred speech
   a. ↓ strength L, slurred speech
   b. c/o weak L side and slurred speech
   c. weakness L side, slurred speech

4. States she has a "splitting" headache
   a. pt. states headache
   b. c/o "splitting" HA
   c. "splitting" HA post assisted ADL

5. Vital signs within normal limits, except for BP @ 180/100
   a. BP ↑ 180/100, TPR no Δ
   b. VS WNL, except BP to 180/100
   c. BP ↑ from 150/88 to 180/100, VS normal range

The exercise demonstrates that there are different ways to express the same information; it is the syntax, and the brevity of the correct answer, that makes it preferable. The syntax, the way the words are arranged leaves little room for misunderstanding the information. Syntax is an important tool to help caregivers decrease the potential for error.

CONTEXT: ACTUAL AND POTENTIAL PROBLEMS

The data that you chart consist of reportable facts that are actual or real. Do not chart potential problems or the rationale for assessing for potential problems. While you may be considering how to document the pathophysiology in terms of "potential for," this information belongs in the *context* of preventable complications in your care plan or pathway. For instance, your patient may be "at

---

BOX 4.3

Improper English

Letting go of formal sentence structure can be difficult. We have been taught that clear thoughts depend on the proper use of the parts of a sentence. We have all been humiliated by dangling participles and the offensive "end of sentence" preposition.

Now you are learning another way to write and speak. You are learning to write and speak and *think* in shorthand. In clinical situations, in which seconds make a difference, we rely on each other to interpret brief "messages" that are sent in code.

For instance, if you are asked to "prep the patient for surgery STAT," you do not have time to ask for a detailed list of expected actions. Your response becomes automatic. You prepare the patient physically, psychologically, and legally for surgery as thoroughly as possible considering the "stat" order.

You will find this holds true for many of your daily activities. It seems like an impossible task to retain all the information needed to decode one word or one phrase. However, learning to process the words, the language, gradually through your education will help.

---

risk for" fluid volume deficit. The desired outcome is adequate hydration. The pathophysiology might be outlined as "NPO $\rightarrow \downarrow$ fluid intake $\rightarrow \downarrow$ fluid volume or fluid volume deficit/hypovolemia." This is the rationale for the order to deliver IV fluids at 1000 cc/8 hr shift.

The record should reflect the action, fluid delivery, and the physical manifestations that support its effectiveness. Do not include a rationale in your written report. The "potential problem" is not a factual notation.

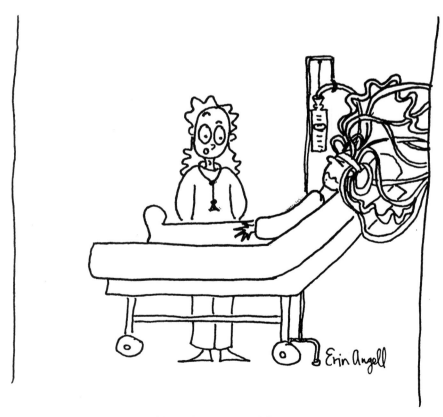

Bad hair day, potential for . . . .

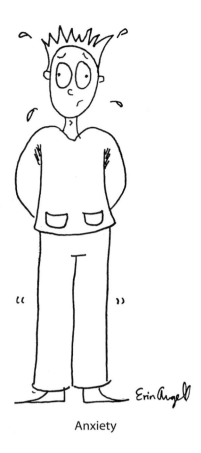

Anxiety

In the correct context, such as the care plan or pathway, the nursing diagnosis that acknowledges the "potential problem" is a prompt to help staff members maintain awareness of all possibilities. It is a reminder to be watchful for early indicators of a problem, even as you are focusing on actual problems.

Figure 4.2

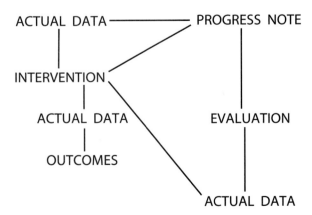

Progress notes contain real or actual data. Real data reflect the actual status of the patient. Real data support intervention. Interventions are documented. Outcomes (subjective and objective) of interventions are documented. Outcomes are evaluated and assessed to determine their effectiveness. Actual or real data reflect the current status of the patient.

Factual data are recorded in the patient's flow chart and progress record. In the case of "potential for fluid volume deficit," a patient record showing "weight loss, dry mucous membranes, increased temperature, decreased urine output, and increased specific gravity" reflects real, or actual, data that support changing your nursing diagnosis from potential to actual. Nursing interventions are then altered from the prevention of a potential problem to restoration of fluid balance. Further changes in the objective parameters then reflect the effectiveness of the interventions.

Content, or information, is organized to promote clarity. Within your format you have the tools to present clear contextual data.

INTEGRATING INFORMATION

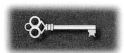

You are learning to integrate your theoretical knowledge base and your technical skills. You can see how understanding the subtle and not so subtle uses of language assists in meeting this daily challenge. As you understand the words associated with nursing's technical language, and how they are used in terms of format, context and syntax, you will be able to problem solve which implied nursing actions will likely result in the desired outcomes.

In integrating your theoretical and functional knowledge, you consider the possible interventions and the rationale for the interventions to report to your instructor. You then suggest a plan of care as well as a scheme for time management. Your planning is completed prior to seeing the patient. Data from your first interview are used to individualize nursing care to meet the patient's needs. Concurrent diagnoses are prioritized along with psychosocial factors, which may influence the patient's response to care.

Case Study 4.3

Patient M is a 45 y/o, white, male about to be admitted to your unit for a bowel obstruction secondary to chronic diverticulitis. Colonoscopy reveals near-complete obstruction of the descending colon. The patient complains of severe abdominal pain, intermittent nausea and vomiting, and small amounts of thin ribbon stool times six days. T 101°F, there is a noticeable loss of appetite, an inability to retain fluids, and decreased urine output.

You are preparing for your clinical day and have an instructor who practices the Socratic instructional technique. You expect questions such as "What does that mean to you?" and "What interventions might you plan?"

BOX 4.4

Possible Interventions

NPO
NG to low suction
TPN (central line)
IV fluid replacement
Pain assessment and control (PCA)
I & O
VS

None of the above were mentioned in the case study. All of the above are likely interventions for bowel obstruction.

Your ability to understand language, and to assess what is implied in that language allows you to establish a basic plan for care, to prepare necessary equipment, and assess hours of care. Time saved can then be dedicated to individualizing care.

LANGUAGE THAT "IMPLIES" ACTION

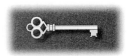

Many technical words characterize a situation, an assessment need, or an action. These words should trigger application of the nursing process. The name of a procedure or a description of a patient's current status implies assessment, prioritization, and possible intervention. You are alerted to potential problems and expected outcomes. As you have seen in reviewing NANDA, nursing care is dependent on your recognizing words that imply action.

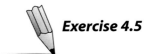 **Exercise 4.5**

Word scramble. Read the words listed. If the word implies action without modifiers, mark "A" or action word. If a modifier can alter a word to imply action, write in the letter of the descriptor from the second list which modifies the meaning. The descriptors can be used more than once. Other words may not be used at all.

1. kidney	A. action word
2. heart	B. obstruction
3. bowel	C. labile
4. unconscious	D. failure
5. embolus	E. abdominal
6. headache	F. attack
7. airway	G. pulmonary
8. obtunded	H. active
9. moribund	I. acute
10. distension	J. compound
11. hemorrhage	K. malignant
12. labor	L. severe
13. cyanosis	M. diabetic
14. malnutrition	N. ileus
15. hypertension	O. hepatic
16. seizure	P. grand mal
17. asthma	Q. kidney
18. coma	R. peritoneal
19. post-op	S. arrhythmia
20. fracture	T. respiratory
21. dialysis	U. arrest
22. hyperthermia	V. precipitous
23. distress	
24. cardiac	

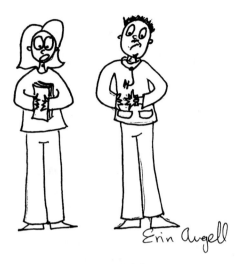

Anxiety, potential for

If a goal is to decrease stress, you need to define what that means and how you will assess the outcome. Recording that the patient "appears calmer" means absolutely nothing to a chart review team.

Read the following phrases and words. Individually they present very few facts. Yet they each are able to create a visual image as well as alert an experienced nurse to observe carefully for potential problems related to that image.

Foley catheter in place

pt arrives to the ED with c/o acute crushing chest pain . . .

moderate to severe respiratory distress

speaks in 1–2 word sentences only

pt. observed to have an apparent lapse of conscious ability to verbally interact to questions, eyes were noted to be deviated upward and to the right.

pt. found to be pulseless and without respiratory effort.

C-section

Post-op

Dialysis

Diabetes

Exercise 4.6

Select the words in each phrase that imply an nursing action or observation. Write possible nursing actions that are implied.

1. Pt unconscious on admit to ER
2. Pt observed to be obtunded
3. Pt restless 48 hours post MI

4. Urinary retention 3 days post C-section
5. Patient admitted in active labor
6. Patient returned to floor after TURP
7. Patient to recovery room post C-section
8. Patient to unit post-op appendectomy
9. Surgical patient with concurrent diagnosis of diabetes
10. Patient to begin kidney dialysis every three days

CREATING THE WORD PICTURE

By learning the technical meaning of words, you will develop a specialized vocabulary for presenting patient data. This in turn is used to create a word picture that communicates the patient's situation to other caregivers. In this way, the nursing process is perpetuated. In nursing education these "word pictures" are known as patient case studies.

Case Study 4.4

Read the case study and following observations.

You are a new graduate nightshift nurse assigned to do primary care of three patients on a medical-surgical (med-surg) unit. Your patients are:

Mr. X, a 55-year-old male, 6 hours post op, transurethral resection of the prostate (TURP) for the primary diagnosis of benign prostatic hypertrophy (BPH).

Mrs. Y, a 37-year-old female visiting family in the area. She experienced a sudden and acute onset of severe, generalized abdominal pain with exquisite tenderness accompanied by nausea and persistent emesis. She was admitted for further observation and monitoring.

Ms. Z, a 28-year-old female with pneumonia. She has a history of asthma, which has required hospitalization and intubation in the past. She was admitted after multiple breathing treatments failed to reduce accessory muscle usage.

At 0400 rounds you make the following observations and assessments:

Mr. X, vital signs stable, patient is alert and oriented to verbal requests, #26 Foley catheter with 30 cc balloon inflated in the bladder and connected to continuous irrigation. The drainage is clear and tinted pink. He is also complaining of pain in his abdominal area. When asked, he says the pain is "mild" and points to the mid-abdomen. He has an IV PCA in place, which he says has been successful in relieving the pain.

Mrs. Y appeared to be sleeping much of the night when you checked, although she did complain of pain in her left lower quadrant, which came intermittently and was rated by Mrs. Y as "3–4" on a pain scale of 1–10. She was also up to the bathroom and voided clear, amber urine. Mrs. Y stated that she had a bowel movement and was pleased that she did not experience pain, even though you had to help her ambulate to the bathroom. Upon inspection, you note that her bowel movement is soft and formed, brown, and no traces of blood are noted.

Ms. Z had some difficulty with congestion and breathing easily when resting flat in her bed. As you listen with your stethoscope, you note wheezing noises in both of her upper lung fields, with each expiration sounding prolonged and labored. She could not seem to get comfortable until the respiratory therapist came and delivered a nebulized air treatment per the physician's PRN order.

After that, you listened to her lungs and noted that the wheezes were resolved. The respiratory therapist tells you that Ms. Z's oxygen saturation pretreatment was 92% and now, posttreatment, it is 98% on room air. Ms. Z seemed much relieved and went back to sleep on her back in bed. As you listened to her breathing from the doorway, you notice that her respirations seem much less labored, the inspiratory phase is equal to the expiratory phase and Ms. Z has no audible evidence of noises with her respirations.

Choose which of the following most clearly creates a concise, complete picture of the observations.

MR. X

A. A/O, #26 Foley with 30 cc balloon to cont sterile water irrig, pink, clear drainage, c/o mild pain low mid-abdomen relieved by PCA.
B. Pt was alert with mild complaint of pain, noted clear, pink, drainage from Foley, states pain relieved when uses PCA for relief
C. Pt had clear, pink, drainage from Foley with sterile water for continuous irrigation, had some pain in lower, middle abdomen but states used PCA successfully, A/O.
D. Pt, c/o mild pain, 6 hrs. post-op in abdomen which was relieved with use of PCA, A/O, with clear, pink drainage from Foley connected to cont. drainage of sterile water.

MRS. Y

A. Pt. s̄ verbal c/o pain when checked hourly thru nite. Respirations even at rest, no acute distress observed/verbalized. Cont c/o intermittent pain, lt. lower quadrant; "3–4" on a pain scale of 10. Up to BR to void clear, amber urine. Pt. reports 1 soft, formed, brown stool, no observable traces blood on visual inspection. Pt. without c/o pain when assisted up to BR.
B. Pt. checked hourly, no pain post assist to BR to void. Urine clear & amber. Pt states 1 stool which was soft and brown and formed. Still c/o occasional pain left side, without it increasing when up to BR with assist. Pain noted to be 3–4 on 1–10 scale. Even respirations while sleeping.
C. Pt. observed to have even respiration at rest, without any c/o pain at rest or up to BR with assist, and which produced 1 formed, soft, brown stool and clear amber urine. Intermittent pain stated as 3–4 out of 10, lt lower abdomen. No acute distress observed.
D. Patient observed to be in no acute distress with pain of 3–4 out of 1–10 scale. Not increased when assisted up to BR for 1 stool which was formed, soft, and brown and to urinate clear amber urine. No blood on stool. Pain was in left lower quadrant. Respirations are even at rest.

MS. Z

A. Pt. with dyspnea and congestion when supine in bed. Bilateral wheezing upper lung lobes with prolonged & labored end expiratory effort. O2 sat 92%, room air. PRN RT treatment via HHN, lungs clear post treatment via auscultation. O2 sat 98%, room air. Pt. settles to resting quiet with no further c/o difficulty. Respirations even at rest, no audible acute distress noted when checked hourly thereafter.

B. Pt noted to be having shortness of breath and congestion while lying flat in bed. Auscultation revealed some bilateral wheezes and expiratory effort. Oximeter revealed O2 sat of 92%. RT to bedside for HHN tx with result of O2 to 98% and relief of difficulty. Quiet respirations with pt. resting comfortably for one hour.

C. RT notified for PRN treatment when pt found to have SOB and wheezing on auscultation esp. while lying flat. Respiratory effort was bilateral with O2 sat of 92% prior to treatment and 98% after. Pt continues to rest post treatment.

D. Pt. admits to dyspnea and congestion when noted to have difficulty while supine. RT notified to do PRN breathing treatment after O2 sat taken at 92%. Post RT treatment pt. end expiratory effort improved and bil wheezes absent in both upper lung lobes via auscultation. Pt resting comfortably with no further complaints when checked one hour after treatment.

Answer Guide

Exercise 4.1

1. alter
   Common: change; tailor; castrate or spay
   Technical: change

2. atraumatic
   Common: no trauma
   Technical: without trauma

3. calf
   Common: young cow
   Technical: muscular area of the lower portion of the leg

4. compress
   Common: condense
   Technical: pads or gauze applied for pressure, heat, or cold

5. deficit
   Common: shortfall of money; inadequate
   Technical: insufficient; that which is being consumed faster than replaced

6. implant
   Common: to set firmly; instill
   Technical: graft; insert in tissue; put in surgically

7. incontinent
   Common: not controlled; unable to be restrained
   Technical: unable to control excretory functions

8. invasive
   Common: denoting an the act of violating; tending to overrun harmfully
   Technical: denoting a puncture, incision, or penetration of the body; relating to the spread of neoplasm to adjoining tissue

9. main
   Common: most important; large pipe or conduit
   Technical: primary source, such as coronary arteries

10. met
    Common: past tense of the word *meet*
    Technical: shortened form of the word *metastasis* (spread or implant of neoplasm to other tissue)

11. morbid
    Common: gruesome, grisly; unwholesome preoccupation
    Technical: related to disease; deviant

12. moribund
    Common: near death
    Technical: dying; death imminent

13. needleless
    Common: no needle
    Technical: any system which has been modified to eliminate needle use

14. potential
    Common: latent; expected capacity for development
    Technical: possible but not real; action which may take place under proscribed conditions

15. status
    Common: legal definition of state of person or thing; high social regard
    Technical: condition; assessment of patient state

16. trauma
    Common: wound or war shock
    Technical: wound or shock; injury accidental or purposefully inflicted

17. tube
    Common: pipe; hollow cylinder
    Technical: canal; hollow organ; or any pipe through which oxygen, medication, or food is given, or fluid drained from body orifice

18. valve
    Common: structure which regulates the flow of gas or liquid
    Technical: membrane of canal or hollow organ that prevents reflux of fluid

19. impaired
    Common: diminished; harmed
    Technical: weakened; damaged; deteriorated

20. intolerance
    Common: unbearable nature; bigotry
    Technical: inability to handle substance or inability to endure

21. obtunded
    Common: oblivious to external stimuli
    Technical: reduced level of consciousness due to analgesia, or use of drugs or alcohol

Exercise 4.2

1. deficit
2. altered
3. impaired
4. risk for
5. intolerance
6. ineffective

7. less than/more than body requirements
8. effective
9. potential for

Exercise 4.3

1. Nutrition, less than body requirements
2. Gas exchange, impaired
3. Airway, ineffective
4. Infection, risk for
5. Protection, altered

Exercise 4.4

1. (C), (I), (I), (I)
2. (C), (A), (A), (A), (I), (I)
3. (O), (A), (A), (I)
4. (C), (I), (O)
5. (I), (C), (A), (A), (A), (I)

Exercise 4.5

1. kidney—(D) failure
2. heart—(F) attack, (D) failure
3. bowel—(B) obstruction
4. unconscious—(A) action word
5. embolus—(G) pulmonary
6. headache—(I) acute, (L) severe
7. airway—(B) obstruction
8. obtunded—(A) action word
9. moribund—(A) action word
10. distension—(E) abdominal
11. hemorrhage—(I) acute, (L) severe
12. labor—(H) active, (V) precipitous
13. cyanosis—(A) action word
14. malnutrition—(A) action word
15. hypertension—(K) malignant, (C) labile
16. seizure—(P) grand mal, (M) diabetic
17. asthma—(I) acute
18. coma—(O) hepatic, (M) diabetic
19. post-op—(A) action word
20. fracture—(J) compound
21. dialysis—(Q) kidney, (R) peritoneal
22. hyperthermia—(K) malignant
23. distress—(T) respiratory
24. cardiac—(S) arrhythmia

Exercise 4.6

1. **Unconscious:** assess status of airway; check for patient pulses; determine support need; initiate CPR if indicated; assess for cause of LOC; initiate O2 assist; contact physician immediately; perform FSBG at bedside; start IV line and consider giving dextrose or Narcan; EKG; ask family members "what happened?"; draw blood for further laboratory analysis; consider possibility of accidental or intentional overdose of substance

2. **Obtunded:** assess and open patient's airway; check pulses; initiate CPR if indicated; reposition patient upright in bed; initiate O2 assist; contact physician immediately; check O2 saturation; perform FSBG at bedside; start IV line and consider giving dextrose or Narcan; EKG; draw blood for laboratory analysis; check medications administered

3. **Restless:** Assess oxygenation, pain; assess for pain; EKG; take vital signs with BP q 5–15 minutes; administer medications per standing orders; draw blood for laboratory analysis; portable chest x-ray; reassess pain; IV medications via bolus or drip to address pain, ectopy, or low BP; cardiology consult

4. **Retention:** prepare for urinary catheterization; assess ease of catheterization or bloody urine return; draw lab to assess for renal function/status; contact patient's primary physician; anticipate possible IVP; monitor vital signs; monitor I & O

5. **Active labor:** assess quality, intensity and timing of uterine contractions; assess if fetus is crowning; assess dilation and effacement of cervix; remind mother not to push until ready to deliver baby; prepare for delivery of the baby; prepare delivery area to receive and resuscitate neonate; contact obstetrician; provide O2 throughout delivery

6. **TURP:** Catheter with 30 cc balloon; observe urine drainage for color, character, consistency, and amount; anticipate patient needs post spinal or general anesthetic; assess pain; discharge teaching to include sexual issues and questions

7. **C-Section:** urinary catheter; post-op ambulation; post-op bowel status; wound precautions and incisional healing; neonatal care integration; pain and comfort interventions; numerous visitors

8. **Post-Op:** altered or diminished consciousness; frequent vital sign monitoring; assess level of mentation and orientation; pain assessment; initiate turn, cough, and deep breathe regimen; potential for nausea and emesis; IV fluid needs; assist to bathroom; physician notification regarding status change; surgical wound considerations and care needs

9. **Diabetes:** need for insulin; frequency of FSBG; circulation checks; dietary considerations; lifelong need for education; lifestyle accommodations and changes; family support structure; discharge planning and teaching needs; patient/family familiarity with signs of hyper- and hypoglycemia

10. **Dialysis:** patient access shunt; skin checks; lifelong need for education; lifestyle accommodations and changes; family support structure; discharge planning and teaching needs; fluid intake and output concerns; dietary restrictions; dialysis schedule and emergency care plan; infection control issues

Case Study 4.2
1. c
2. c
3. c
4. b
5. a

Case Study 4.4
Mr X: A
Mrs. Y: A
Ms. Z: A

CHAPTER 5

Managing Bias in Documentation

This chapter will help you to differentiate between the subjective and objective characteristics of patient assessment data. You will also learn ways to include relevant information in the written record or verbal report. The focus is on the observation and inclusion of pertinent data related to the patient, a chief complaint or system assessment. You will also be introduced to the concept of bias in the form of words or actions related a patient's health assessment, status, or history.

The SOAP charting and CHH/ROS formats both require a nurse to clearly understand and document the differences between subjective and objective information obtained from the patient. A novice nurse who is not comfortable with the responsibility of this task may find charting a difficult assignment. The teaching content in this chapter clarifies the important distinction between objective and subjective data.

WORD LIST

complaint	decline	refuse
deviant	radiation	obese
character	discipline	cretin
bias	insipid	expel
objective	vapid	incompetence
subjective	indolent	ordinary
compliant	noncompliant	irreversible
failure		

 Exercise 5.1

Each item in the word list has both common and technical meanings. Match each word with its corresponding set of definitions and compare the intent or usage of the terms as both common and technical words.

1. _____
   Common: traits that define a person's integrity or behavior; a shorthand symbol that represents a value of some description; slang that portrays behavior as interesting and singular
   Technical: traits that describe in detail a specific complaint or symptom

2. _____
   Common: refuse; reject; descend
   Technical: refuse; to deteriorate in condition

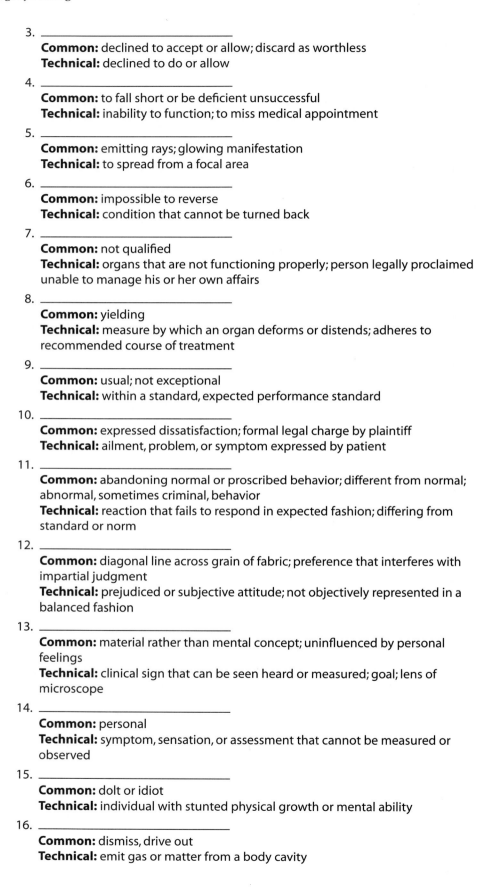

3. _____
Common: declined to accept or allow; discard as worthless
Technical: declined to do or allow

4. _____
Common: to fall short or be deficient unsuccessful
Technical: inability to function; to miss medical appointment

5. _____
Common: emitting rays; glowing manifestation
Technical: to spread from a focal area

6. _____
Common: impossible to reverse
Technical: condition that cannot be turned back

7. _____
Common: not qualified
Technical: organs that are not functioning properly; person legally proclaimed unable to manage his or her own affairs

8. _____
Common: yielding
Technical: measure by which an organ deforms or distends; adheres to recommended course of treatment

9. _____
Common: usual; not exceptional
Technical: within a standard, expected performance standard

10. _____
Common: expressed dissatisfaction; formal legal charge by plaintiff
Technical: ailment, problem, or symptom expressed by patient

11. _____
Common: abandoning normal or proscribed behavior; different from normal; abnormal, sometimes criminal, behavior
Technical: reaction that fails to respond in expected fashion; differing from standard or norm

12. _____
Common: diagonal line across grain of fabric; preference that interferes with impartial judgment
Technical: prejudiced or subjective attitude; not objectively represented in a balanced fashion

13. _____
Common: material rather than mental concept; uninfluenced by personal feelings
Technical: clinical sign that can be seen heard or measured; goal; lens of microscope

14. _____
Common: personal
Technical: symptom, sensation, or assessment that cannot be measured or observed

15. _____
Common: dolt or idiot
Technical: individual with stunted physical growth or mental ability

16. _____
Common: dismiss, drive out
Technical: emit gas or matter from a body cavity

17. _____

    Common: punishment; training for strict order or behavior
    Technical: specific medical specialty

18. _____

    Common: lazy
    Technical: not active; not an active medical problem

19. _____

    Common: dull; without flavor or tasteless
    Technical: not arousing interest; vague

20. _____

    Common: not malleable
    Technical: not able or willing to comply with treatment regimen

21. _____

    Common: extremely overweight
    Technical: abnormally overweight by a defined percentage.

22. _____

    Common: not interested; not lively
    Technical: dull; listless

THE DIFFERENCE BETWEEN SUBJECTIVE AND OBJECTIVE DATA

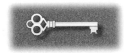

Your task is to learn to differentiate between subjective and objective data. In other words, you need to understand what patient-based information is pertinent, when it is included in a patient's record, how to record it in a legal manner, and if the information reveals caregiver bias.

Objective data include clear, descriptive content. The information has measurable parameters or outcomes. The nurse may employ a critical thinking process to lead to assessment of available data using useful problem solving techniques, and then record that assessment in professional, minimally biased language.

Disease diagnosis and a patient's personal health habits can raise bias on the part of the health practitioner. Have you ever wondered why the patient with chronic lung disease is also a smoker? How about the patient with gallbladder disease who eats fried, fatty foods? Words trigger emotion in patients *and* caregivers. For example, consider the impact of these statements: "grossly obese"; "positive for HIV status"; or "liver cancer with metastasis to the brain." Your careful and professional selection of language both in the medical record and in communicating with co-workers will help to minimize misinformation and bias.

Generally, much of the data you collect is subjective information obtained from the patient. Your learning task is to objectively differentiate within the subjective information set and to organize it in a consistent manner, between different caregivers. There are documentation tools to help you in this endeavor. Checklists almost automatically clarify your assessments. Policies and standards for documentation at your place of employment are also available. Wherever possible, scales have been devised to describe and quantify assessment data. Some examples include the Glasgow Coma Score; the Wong-Baker facies pain scale for children; and a patient determined pain rating system from 1–5 or 1–10.

If you are a novice, now is the time to develop some working habits. An excellent skill is that of always asking for help when you are unsure. Also, complete all parts of a form rather than leaving portions blank. "Not applicable" (N/A) is acceptable if information is not available at the time. "Unknown" or "not stated" is also acceptable if the patient is unable to provide an answer.

If you do want to include a patient's subjective remarks in the medical record, place the statement in direct quotation marks to indicate the legal source of origin. *Remember, we are not required to have all the answers; rather, we are simply required to legally and professionally note what was or was not able to be obtained from a patient history or examination at the time of your inquiry.*

SUBJECTIVE DATA AND BIAS WORDS

Where in health care does bias come from? Consider this. Subjective data is based upon personal interpretation (by the patient or the caregiver) of information that by its nature may be difficult to measure precisely. It is true that we have tools with which to record the tangible signs of illness such as vital signs, blood chemistries, lung sounds, and other observable parameters of a patient's status. There are, however, many physical manifestations that do not have exact criteria or systems to standardize measurement between practitioners.

Pain is one such manifestation. It is a primary symptom that involves inexact and inconsistent measurements for assessment. Each patient has an individual response level, or tolerance for pain. Caregivers make use of pain measurement techniques such as Wong-Baker facies and numerical scales to interpret each patient's pain response. As a nurse, you have no control over the patient's individualized perception of their own pain. It is therefore necessary to be consistent in the description of a patient's pain level. You may create your own uniform parameters that translate into "mild, moderate, severe, and exquisite" levels of pain, but you must be aware of the bias you are creating within your measurement system. As you guide the patient by asking questions about their description of symptoms, remember that just the words "Is the pain sharp or dull?" provide the patient a vocabulary of bias words that have the potential to change how pain level is interpreted by either the patient or the caregiver.

A patient's interpretation of painful symptoms is also based on the patient's level of understanding as well as their prior experience with similar symptoms. Consider the preverbal infant whose parents are worried because the child is not "acting right." The parents are familiar with the child's usual behavior and notice subtle differences that may indicate to them that the child is not feeling well.

A patient who has a history of migraine headaches might compare any subsequent pain against what they understand as the "worst pain" they have experienced with a migraine. In fact, the patient with a positive history of myocardial infarction who presents with a complaint of "chest pain" will be asked if the pain is similar to the pain at the time of the myocardial infarction.

Each patient values pain differently and each patient expresses their *evaluation* of the complaint differently. A patient who has fear of pain may "rate" the slightest pain as very high on the scale. The anticipation of pain may intensify their experience. Nurses document pain according to the patient's interpretation. If the pain is valued at "9 on a scale of 10," how is this response viewed by the nurse?

First, is the pain consistent with the expected pain level associated with the cause? "Expected" in this case, though subjectively determined by the caregiver, is usually supported by medical data and the nurse's experience with the presenting complaint. If the pain is not consistent, the caregiver is obligated to further determine what may be contributing to an unusually high level of pain.

Cultural influences may also alter an individual's interpretation of a symptom. If a patient has been required culturally to withhold complaints or to withstand discomfort without sharing feelings, they may not be prepared to verbalize specific problems.

A patient's age, literacy, and language disparity may also interfere with effective communication between patient and caregiver. You must be prepared to adapt your vocabulary, to speak with interpreters who may have no medical background, and to use nonverbal skills in order to gain accurate information from a patient. Be comfortable with your own knowledge and skills before seeking information from a patient. Look up disease or symptoms with which you are unfamiliar. Find out about cultural differences to understand the patient and review age differences in order to form therapeutic relationships that are effective for you and the patient.

Experience will add to your knowledge base and to your communication skills. Your exposure to various patients or situations will help you to quickly assess the patient's receptivity to an interview and to their ability to respond to questions.

At the same time, be clear about your role and know your own biases. The nurse's ability to communicate is dependent upon listening and language skills.

 Exercise 5.2

Match the subjective word with its more objective equivalent.

1. whining _____	hesitant speech
2. smells bad _____	unable to complete staff requests
3. denies _____	smell of alcohol on breath
4. refuse _____	no permanent residence
5. difficult _____	resting with eyes closed
6. stutter _____	complaint
7. asleep _____	noted to be crying at intervals
8. drunk _____	states no
9. noncompliant _____	poor hygiene
10. homeless _____	decline
11. fussy _____	uncooperative to verbal request
12. possible CVA _____	witnessed loss of motor functions unilaterally

Subjective information is like an overview or outline of a patient complaint or event that needs specific, more precise information to complete the patient's explanation. You need to quantify time frames, amounts, and other measurable data elements as accurately as possible. Each detail will provide the health care team with a better opportunity to address a defined problem rather than a generalized one.

Subjective data are often translated or interpreted by the listener. The interpreter may be the caregiver or someone close to the patient who in turn relays the information. The caregiver then places a value on the data based on past assessment information, the pathophysiology of the problem, and the caregiver's own bias toward the patient or pathology. Data direct from the patient may be interpreted or weighted by the caregiver differently than information shared by family or friends. The caregiver then makes an independent judgment about further assessment and intervention and is placed in a position of "power" over the patient's well-being. This is a sacred trust.

By now you have likely heard the words "active listening." You may even be sick of hearing about the technique. It is necessary to understand the words "active" and "listen" in order to narrow down subjective, patient-based data to

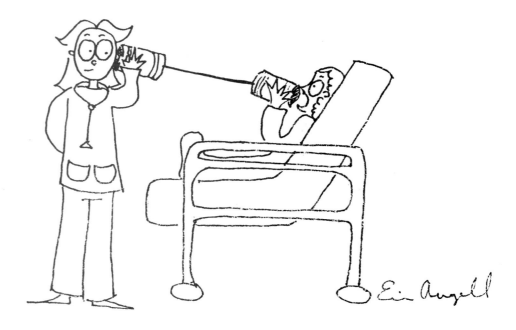

more objective determinations. People process information rapidly and often filter bits of information retaining only what they prioritize. As you listen to a patient's complaint or needs, you have to hear what they are saying and follow up with appropriate questions using language the patient can understand. You have to watch how the patient reacts as well as responds to each inquiry, often needing to determine what the patient means.

Family Input

A patient's family may express their concern about the staff understanding and interpreting a loved one's needs. Listening to family members can yield vital information about the patient's usual response to illness or pain.

For instance, if a family member states, "Mom must be in a lot pain if she is asking for medication," explore the basis for that observation. You may learn that the patient had a three-year history of "remarkable" abdominal discomfort with no significant change in her daily activities.

Many individuals with angina suffer for a prolonged time without diagnosis and are only treated after a major cardiac episode. They may regard symptoms of chest pain as part of their "normal" behavior and disregard the potential until a debilitating event occurs.

On the flip side there are patients who are incapacitated by even the most minor symptomatology. Every sneeze is viewed as an illness and worthy of obsessive attention.

Both types of patients can be problematic because you must vigilantly pay appropriate attention to their needs in spite of possible over- or underreaction by the patient. Family members need to be reassured that you will be vigilant in assessment, that you are experienced in eliciting forthright responses regarding symptoms, and that you will provide the best care possible.

Documentation of all significant data about symptoms is the safeguard and the proof that you have assessed the patient, recorded your findings, and planned your nursing care based on quantifiable data.

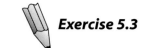

Exercise 5.3

Match the following phrases with possible meanings.

1. I am upset. _____
2. No one is listening to me. _____
3. I am supposed to be ready to go home tomorrow. _____
4. Everything's going to be all right. _____
5. My nurse is mad at me. _____
6. PT says I have to learn how to do this alone. _____
7. I want to know what is wrong with me. _____
8. My doctor doesn't want to give me more pain medicine. _____
9. I might need an operation. _____

A. Patient is expressing that a surgical procedure may be required.

B. Patient is asking for further information or explanation to understand his diagnosis.

C. Patient is expressing verbal concern about a condition or event.

D. Verbal response, often from health care provider, offered in attempt to reassure patient.

E. Patient expresses that the physical therapist is teaching the patient exercise or activity that the patient will learn to perform without assistance.

F. Patient perceives that at least one, possibly more, providers are not affirming to him what he is attempting to express verbally.

G. Patient expresses a perception that his nurse is unhappy or angry with him.

H. Patient may be verbally expressing a hesitation, lack of confidence, or feeling that he is not prepared or capable of discharge from the care facility.

I. Patient is expressing a lack of agreement or understanding regarding the quantity of medication available for his complaints of pain.

WHERE DO BIASES COME FROM?

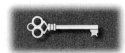

The technical definition for *bias* according to Webster is "an inclination or preference that interferes with impartial judgment: prejudice." While no one is born with bias, it will develop naturally, depending on a person's background, upbringing, and experiences. Bias in itself is not wrong; however, biases can affect how caregivers hear, listen, and interpret subjective data.

Know your own biases toward people, age, ethnicity, or disease processes. The way a person speaks, the words a person uses, literacy levels, even accents, can change how one person is viewed by another. Bias can affect how you care for your patient. Your own subconscious can sway your understanding and subsequent interpretation of the patient's words.

Nurses do not pick and choose their patients. If you are working in a geographic area with few hospitals, your patients will likely represent a cross section of the community. You may see patients who demonstrate all manner of speech, such as slang usage, accents, age-related peculiar speech habits, and ethnic references. You may also observe various styles of body language specific to a patient's comfort level with the health care system.

Caregivers may feel an aversion to a patient because of certain traits. Health habits such as drinking or smoking and idiosyncrasies such as chewing hair, picking at teeth, or scratching can be annoying and even elicit feelings of disgust. A patient's personal habits and choices may often cause our biases to surface.

For example, smoking is a health habit reviled by many health care workers, who may even blame patients who smoke for their illness. They may focus on the patient's smoking without regard to the patient's immediate complaint, even if unrelated to the smoking history. Other personal habits can cause bias and irritate or annoy an observer, such as scratching, finger tapping, facial tics, or nervous speech habits.

Illness that is considered to be preventable, such as lung cancer, AIDS, or STDs, can cause the nurse to form value judgments. Nurses have shown bias against patients with certain health problems. Smoking-related pulmonary disease and AIDS are two that are very difficult for many caregivers to work with.

BOX 5.2

On Being "Politically Correct"

Language is being scrutinized as never before to determine if individuals are being discriminated against due to bias. As nurses, you will be committing your interpretation of patient interviews in writing for use by the health care team in planning care. You do not anticipate that each statement may be reviewed and interpreted based on the "legal" definition of terms. However, you and your patients will benefit if you document with the awareness that all notes have the potential to be litigated.

As you choose your descriptive terms, be cognizant of the impact these words may have on anyone who might be reviewing your chart. We have discussed the importance of correctly referencing race and ethnic origin. You may need to ask your patient how they define their ethnic origin. Your work setting should have a policy related to race as well as to statements about ethnicity. Follow that policy. If the policy has the potential to promote bias or is offensive, be proactive in suggesting that the policy might be rewritten to reflect less bias.

If you are documenting a patient's health habits, lifestyle choices, and appearance, be aware that words commonly used in a hospital environment may be subject to interpretation by those who know only the common definition. Descriptors such as "noncompliant" and "noncooperative" can be skewed to sound like you are faulting a patient if not viewed in the context of the noted event.

Imagine a written note documenting patient contact with a combative IV drug user who is homeless, being treated for TB, and has presented to a clinic or emergency room after assaulting a police officer while under the influence of an illegal substance. Valid charting about hygiene (odoriferous), nutrition (cachectic), compliance with TB prescription medications (noncompliant), and violent behavior (hostile and uncooperative) might be interpreted as a nurse using value judgment about a self-destructive patient.

Care needs to be taken in documenting valid information about economic status, weight disorders, and suspected abuse. We all intend to treat patients with equal care and respect but we are human beings who have personal experiences that create bias. Transmitting these biases in a manner that affects care is not appropriate.

You will not be perfect in avoiding biased and politically "incorrect" language. English is a fluid language. The word "gay" used to mean "carefree and happy," a "joint" could be "a place to meet," "an articulation point," or "marijuana," and a reference to a "nurse" always meant the RN. "Ms." is now commonly used, but many women would be offended by this salutation.

It is not important what your personal beliefs are regarding the move toward politically inoffensive speech. It is important that your documentation reflect factual data clearly and be justified according to the technical use of language acceptable in nursing according to the standards in your work setting.

A nurse's own life experience and experiential memories, either good or bad, can influence their response to an individual. In many cases injury or illness are related to a situation. Patients may often remind us of an individual or an experience with which we are uncomfortable. When we are confronted with situations that remind us of a personal experience, either positively or negatively, we are at risk of showing bias. Feelings based on past experience may also influence a nurse's reaction, even if he or she is unaware of a bias.

Patients with cultural, class, educational, or life experience different from that of the caregiver can create subtle reactions, such as fear or anger. A nurse's response to information from that source can easily be subject to a bias based on personal judgment.

Patients who are in an economic class different from our own can bias our interpretation of data or our ability to treat the information objectively. Subcultures that may cause fear and class bias are ethnicity, or poverty, extreme wealth, or less obviously subtle responses toward the less educated blue-collar worker, the "biker," or the elderly patient.

If an interpreter is used, the information is already filtered through one level of translation before the nurse even hears it. Watching the patient while he or she is speaking becomes especially important to ensure the best opportunity to understand what the patient says or means.

Nurses may be less likely to respond to an individual whose personal hygiene is unlike their own or who is less approachable due to offensive odors or appearance.

Judging a patient's behavior or personal habits on moral grounds makes it difficult to make unbiased decisions regarding care. The caregiver may decide that the person's behavior is responsible for the health problem and give the complaint or history less credibility than he or she would to a less offensive patient.

Nurses may have personal biases related to their own religious beliefs or a patient's religious beliefs. For instance, religious orientation may easily bias a nurse against caring for the young, unwed patient requesting an abortion. Value judgments can interfere with sound, objective treatment and care. It may also prejudice the ability to honor a patient's right to participate in health care decisions.

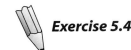

Exercise 5.4

Match from the list a less biased and more accurate description for the following words or statements.

1. poor hygiene _____
2. bad stutter _____
3. disease _____
4. old _____
5. cultural bias _____
6. race _____
7. class _____
8. morals _____
9. religious _____
10. educational level _____

statement indicating someone's declared orientation to religious preference or that someone espouses theologically based values

age stated in years

subjectively based determination of one's financial, social, or economical status

language pattern reflecting repetitive speech habits and difficulty with pronunciation of certain words

evidence of pathological process affecting state of wellness

potential expressed for a predetermined opinion relating to one's cultural orientation

statement indicating an individual's degree or level of formal education ethnicity

foul smelling odor, hair matted, unkempt appearance, shoes worn without socks

ethical or religious opinion, judgment, determination, or value

SUBJECTIVE: QUOTABLE INFORMATION

The subjective data expected in the SOAP format, in the chief complaint for CHH, or in the patient admitting history is the use of the patient's own words to describe the reason he or she is at the clinic or hospital. (This applies to any health care contact.) The patient's response is presented in quotation marks and is not amended by the caregiver or interviewer.

INFLAMMATORY WORDS OR JUDGMENT STATEMENTS

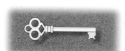

Language is powerful. Words are used to solicit and dispense information. Words can silence or influence the patient guided by the interviewing nurse or provider. Terms such as "tumor," "growth," and "malignant" can frighten a patient and cause them to withdraw or to interpret all further discussion based on their own understanding or personal experience. Words may recall every neighbor's personal horror story and have the potential for great impact on the patient.

Judgmental language spoken to or about a patient can influence whether the patient is heard or even believed by a health care team. Commonly used words to describe patient behavior, "compliant," "uncooperative," "angry," "abusive," "good," "sweet," or "arrogant" are poor descriptors but can carry a heavy impact. A patient's profession, such as lawyer, priest, or convict, may change a caregiver's response to them. The type of insurance coverage can influence a caregiver, particularly if they have strong beliefs about patients who are dependent on government assistance.

Words can easily be misinterpreted. Subjective words that give broad information, without including an objective and measurable descriptor, are especially problematic. For instance, descriptors such as "copious" without a precise measurement, or "frequent" without a numerical account can often mean different things to different caregivers.

Exercise 5.5

In the following statements, circle the word or words that carry increased potential for inflammatory or judgmental language usage.

1. The physician came into the room and said he had seen a tumor on the CAT scan.
2. The man noticed a growth underneath his tongue and wondered about his pipe smoking habit.
3. After a biopsy, the pathologist informed the woman that he thought she had a malignancy. She immediately thought of inoperable cancer.
4. When the nurse asked if the patient had any relevant history of alcohol intake, the patient strongly denied regular alcohol intake or that he considered himself to be an alcoholic or a drunk.
5. He was somewhat uncooperative with the history taking process and, when asked, refused to permit the examination.
6. The doctor informed her that it would be only a minor surgery.
7. The physician noted that the patient showed abusive behaviors, was belligerent and noncompliant to any suggestions.
8. The nurse reported that the patient was homeless, had terrible hygiene and acted illiterate.
9. The older woman came in and began acting bizarre and must have been demented.
10. He was handicapped and therefore obviously disabled.

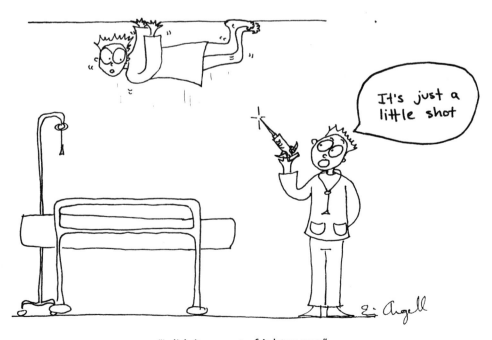

"I didn't mean to frighten you"

OBJECTIVE ONLY

Other than quoted remarks, subjective comments do not belong in your nursing notes. No matter how you feel about a given situation, feelings are not relevant data. For instance, if you are charting a phone call from a doctor that was not returned promptly, simply record time and pertinent information. Even if you want to say that the MD "finally" called, it will not read as intended. It has the potential for insurance or legal interpretations that may be problematic. "Feelings" expressed about "difficult" patients is another area in which any frustration is best expressed somewhere besides the written record.

Charting is not creative writing and notes should not reflect the author's personality. An individual style of expression is not necessarily valued in any legal record recording a patient's care. Notes should be written clearly, concisely, and as close to a standardized format as possible. The only reflection of an individual provider should be in handwriting recognition and signature.

Adjectives can be problematic and must reflect relevancy toward the patient or event. Use of adjectives and descriptors is confined to only those necessary to characterize a problem. Your legal documentation does not require decoration or flourish. Factual information relevant to a patient's diagnosis, treatment, and evaluation is adequate. It is tempting to be creative with descriptors when documenting indicators of a patient's state of mind or complaint of pain. It may also be easy to include adjectives that create a story around a patient's behavior, response to treatment, or psychosocial needs. Nevertheless, restrict your choice of language to "the facts and nothing but the facts" in the event your record is subject to legal review.

Assumptions are dangerous. Do not jump to conclusions when you chart. For example, if you are describing manifestations of probable fluid deficit, avoid conclusions such as "dehydration." You are not licensed to draw conclusions, to make medical diagnoses. Document all physical findings with factual data that

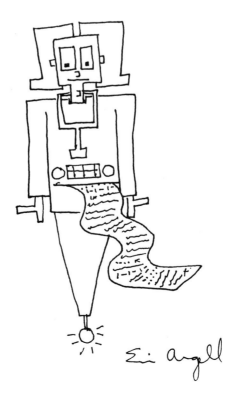

support any suspicions you may have regarding a patient's status, but avoid documenting the assumption itself.

NURSING DIAGNOSES: A FACTUAL DATA BASE

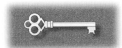

Document all factual data that could assist in drawing a conclusion or making a nursing diagnosis (ND). For instance, consider the patient who states he is "fine" but is grimacing and clutching at his chest. These visible markers seem to conflict with the patient's subjective statement. Other observations could include that his skin is pale and diaphoretic, and that he has an increased heart rate and an elevated blood pressure. Now you have measurable data that lead to nursing-based conclusions. You can act upon and chart this kind of information. Judgment is part of your job and health care decision-making depends upon well-documented, quantified assessment. Data should provide a chronology that allows a medical provider to make medical decisions and for you to make nursing decisions and implement a plan for care.

Data are actual or they are not. Charting is factual or not. Beginning your note with "Patient appears to . . ." may give the impression that you are somehow unsure of your assessment or unable to factually support your determination. Be prepared to be specific in your note. Blood pressure is never "around 120/80." It is "120/80" or it is not. The patient who "seems" to be "in pain" or "looks" asleep is neither in a medical or legal review.

If a measurement is approximated, such as assessing a blood-saturated dressing or urine-soaked sheets, your estimates must be based on the usual amounts that would cause a particular saturation level. Such "guesses" are still only approximate values, but are based on experience. Fluid output measurements such as those from drainage collectors are presented exactly, not as "almost" or "about."

VALUE JUDGMENTS AND RELATED LANGUAGE

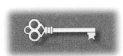

Individual words can trigger emotion. Such terms are commonly used by medical personnel who must be careful to avoid a judgmental effect. For instance the use of *noncompliant* medically indicates that a patient is not adhering to a suggested treatment plan. It may also trigger a sense that the patient is "intentionally" resisting the plan, as in a more common interpretation inferred by the word. It should not be used to suggest any intention on the part of the patient.

BOX 5.3

Negative Words

The following words can all potentially trigger negative impressions and should be used carefully. Use supporting, factual data to amend them as necessary and to avoid judgmental reactions.

- noncompliant
- deviant
- noncooperative
- demented
- unwilling
- refused
- failed

- denied
- combative
- agitated
- inattentive
- illiterate
- malodorous
- nonhygienic
- hostile
- aggressive (aggressive management is a style of treatment; aggressive behavior is unacceptable)
- obese

Many terms may poorly describe patients in a judgmental manner. Some of the familiar, slang-related terms for patients are GOMER (get out of my emergency room), lunger, frequent flyer, vegged out, gorked, or circling the drain.

Many medical professionals are guilty of using these terms to refer to an individual type of patient. These colloquialisms should never find their way into written form. If you find yourself using such slang remember you are referring to your patients, who are depending on you. This level of disrespect undermines your professionalism.

IMPROVING THE STANDARD: USING OBJECTIVE WORDS

Objective data might seem easier to define. This is especially true with data that can be measured with tools and has clinically accepted parameters of "normal." Many observations that seem, at first, to be purely subjective can be described in detail, with experience, using objective terminology. To improve your own abilities, learn bias words and exclude them from your charting unless completely relevant. Make adjectives mean something. Observe and include only relevant data in your written record.

MEASURABLE: MAKING AND KEEPING THE STANDARD

Measurable data are considered objective data. By *measurable* we tend to think of numeric parameters, which also apply here. There are criteria and systems available that allow us to objectively measure, in some cases, a patient's sounds and sensations, for instance, pain scales of 1–10 or heart murmurs scales of 1–6. We can also apply specialized criteria to a problem and draw a measured conclusion. This is true if a specific number of criteria apply in order to reach a conclusion that has relevancy that can be supported by your assessment. An example is the criteria for conversion from HIV status to AIDS, or the criteria applied to a patient that provides the basis for a nursing diagnosis such as fluid deficit or risk for falls.

STANDARDIZING MEANINGS WITH MINIMAL VARIATIONS

There are criteria used to determine objective standards for subjective assessments. The criteria for distinguishing the levels of a heart murmur are clear. They are interpreted only with potential for slight variation among practitioners. It is likely, however, that the variation is not significant, that in fact there may be disagreement with one degree of difference based upon a practitioner's expertise. As long as the practitioner defines his or her own individual range of "normal" consistently, the slight variances among health care personnel is not generally a great problem.

MEASUREMENTS DEFINED CONSISTENTLY

An individual practitioner's consistency is critical. Once a nurse establishes parameters, associates become familiar with the practitioner's judgment, compare it to their own determinations, and by doing so, establish a baseline for evaluation. As individual consistency is developed, one can interpret, within a minor degree of difference, the value of the data being recorded. Consistency in assessment and measurement establishes a reliable basis for dependability. Any

---

BOX 5.4

Common Measurement Techniques

It is common to use a number scale such as 1–5 or 1–10 to assist the patient in quantifying a symptom. You will document this information using a fraction "1/5," and defining your scale "1–5". Choose a scale to use (or use the scale preferred by the facility) and don't deviate. If you always use "1–5" or "1–10" you will avoid errors in your charting.

Murmurs are graded by a set scale of "1–6" written in fraction form. The interpretation of "3/6" or "4/6" may vary slightly among care providers based on experience or hearing ability. There should not be a large variance among providers. If a wide variance is noted it is possible that more than one grade of murmur is present.

Anterior depth of the eye chamber, reflex measurement, and edema are usually graded on a +1–+4 scale with normal predetermined, as with +2 for normal reflex. Size charts are available for determining pupil dilation.

Monitors are used to determine length of a contraction for a woman in labor, recording strength and duration.

The cervical dilation scale is determined in centimeters but is often reported by stating the number of fingers it is possible to insert. This is subject to the variation in hand size but each examiner can determine how many of their own fingers equals each of the parameters on the chart.

Wounds, bruises, skin lesions, and rashes are measured in millimeters or centimeters on the vertical as well as horizontal planes. Raised lesions or swelling may include a measurement of the height from the unaffected skin surface. Photographs are sometimes useful to show progress, either improvement or worsening, of an affected area. Picture documentation should include patient identification in the picture and a measurement device used for showing the scale. Pictures do not take the place of written documentation. They supplement your written data.

Swelling may also be measured for accurate documentation. Abdominal girth is important in determining successful therapy. Measuring edematous extremities provides an exact evaluation tool for therapeutic intervention. If no better measurement is available you can determine changes in edema by the way a patient's shoes or waistbands fit.

Breathing difficulties can be measured by documenting the number of pillows a patient requires for restful sleep. Measure activity by the distance they can walk without breathlessness or fatigue. Stair climbing can also be used to measure fatigue, as well as recovery from certain surgeries, or successful therapy for many forms of arthritis.

---

change in the patient's status is referenced against the patient's "usual" status. Consistent and standardized documentation presented in an objective manner, even of subjectively based assessment, will demonstrate the legal basis for your care.

MEASUREMENTS WITHIN ESTABLISHED PARAMETERS

Work to define your own parameters, your own system, with which to assess the patient's subjective symptoms most objectively. Sometimes there may be associated physical findings that will help you define the parameters. You can also look for groups of symptoms or related data to determine if a patient qualifies for a specific nursing diagnosis.

Related data is also helpful as you work to define pain levels and anxiety, which are not necessarily objective and cannot be so easily measured. Be critical of what you observe. Look for criteria that will help determine the assessed factor objectively. Learn to do this through experience and from instructors or co-workers you value as mentors. By comparing and contrasting your own findings you will learn to establish a level of consistency and relevancy within accepted ranges as well as relate physical findings to the patient's more subjective complaints.

USING DATA TO SUPPORT THE LESS TANGIBLE

Whenever possible reinforce your nursing assessment with measured data from your professional observations. If you write that a patient is "anxious" about surgery, support it with the observable physical manifestations of anxiety such as increased heart rate, sweating, pacing, or nail biting. Such supportive data allow the reader to "see" the patient's behavior. Demonstrate through your documentation that you are not making assumptions and that your assessment of the patient's anxiety is not frivolous or exaggerated. Set scales of measurement, whenever possible, using the same reference scale each time.

If independent practitioners reach the same conclusion each time based on their own assessment of the patient with a subjective complaint, then that data set is more likely to be accurate. Staying objective about patients who are difficult to care for may make objective observation more difficult. Asking for help is especially important if you are having difficulty maintaining a nonjudgmental position with a patient.

Describe actual behavior rather than the effect of the behavior and avoid interpretations of the patient's behavior (Box 5.5). If you are careful to support your assessment with objective observations, you are less likely to simply document your feelings about the behavior. For instance, the statement "smells like he never bathes" may make the patient sound repulsive. "Poor hygiene" presented as a problem within a suggested health teaching context is far less inflammatory.

BOX 5.5

Compare the poor and/or judgmental documentation with the objective, nonbiased counterpart in the following table.

JUDGMENTAL	NONBIASED
Unkempt, dirty, with odor of garbage on ragged clothes	Poor hygiene
Short, withered, unhappy with all attempts at teaching	Frail
Profuse, foul-smelling, bloody diarrhea	475 ml hematochezia
Child was swarming with head lice and scabs from uncontrolled scratching	+head lice, pruritis, crusty lesions mid-occipital, L post auricular, R temporal
Pt. sneaking cigarettes with visitors	Tobacco smoke odor in room

---

MEASURE AS MUCH AS YOU CAN

Any data that can be placed within a measured context should be. Measurable data are evaluated more accurately. This is especially important when planning care for case reviews and quality assurance purposes. It is also a means for ensuring more appropriate reimbursement. Insurance providers will withhold payment if they cannot see documentation supporting results, outcomes, or diagnoses. Record physical manifestations that reinforce vague patient complaints,

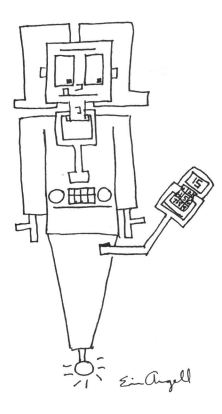

such as anxiety and fear. Patients with cardiac and respiratory ailments frequently have vague, subjective symptoms that need appropriate, supportive data. Consistent observational skills combined with appropriate descriptive documentation are vital to the care of your patients.

THINKING WITH A LINEAR, SYMMETRICAL PERSPECTIVE

Data with exact numerical parameters can easily be charted. To chart subjective data in a linear and objective manner try thinking mathematically. Comparative or symmetrical scales are used successfully with many of our more subjective assessments. Consider, for example, eye exams. If asked to assess the clarity of the lens, compare the left eye with the right eye. Translating your assessments by using comparative language can be very helpful. If assessing dizziness, you can locate in which position (lying, sitting, or standing) the patient is most comfortable and in which position the patient is most distressed. These are mathematical comparisons and ratios. A is to B as C is to D. In this case however A, B, C, and D are contrasted with their own symmetrical value rather than any numerical value.

NORMAL: DIFFERENT AMONG INDIVIDUALS

Individuals relate to feelings in their own individual and subjective way. Pain tolerance, stress reactions, and crisis response are all examples of situations in which a person's background and life experiences may well influence their physical responses. Chronic pain patients live daily with pain levels that might easily be intolerable to one who has not had any prior or extensive pain experience. Patients who are fearful of medical problems may respond with a more

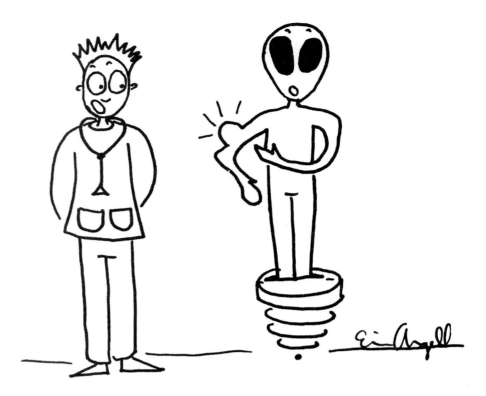

dramatic response than another patient. Their "normal" is not the same as another patient. Nor is it necessarily the same as their caregiver's. We can only work within the patient's own definition and understanding of normal. Be consistent when developing your own sense of "normal" limits or ranges, regarding both the responses you may personally experience or those of a patient you are assessing.

For example, a patient gives an "8/10" in response to your inquiry about the pain experienced. Even if the numerical response is inconsistent with what you would determine to be an "expected" pain level, "8/10" is their interpretation of pain compared to their understanding of "normal" or "no pain." They are not necessarily exaggerating. It may be easy to be judgmental or less sympathetic with these patients. Your nursing care and charting, however, need to remain objective and not reflect your feelings about the patient's response.

USING YOUR SENSES AS OBJECTIVE TOOLS AND HELPMATES

You use sensory tools to provide you with objective data about your patient. You record what you see or hear. Slight facial movements, body language, expression, or attentiveness are all observable attributes about a patient. They describe physical responses. Listen and observe the patient carefully and avoid bias. Ask a patient to clarify and validate what they are saying or what you think you are hearing. Ask them what their words or actions mean to them, because this may often reflect differences in gender, age, or cultures.

Your sense of smell is vital. If you smell alcohol on the driver involved in a motor vehicle accident, semen on a rape victim, or the distinctive aroma of decaying flesh in gangrene, these data are critical and definitive.

Appropriate, professional use of touch can alert you to a patient's body temperature, tone, or moisture changes. It can also help pinpoint pain origin or location of swelling. Touch can easily alert an experienced nurse to early thrombophlebitis, IV infiltration, or inflammation. These observations are then recorded objectively as physical manifestations, using groups of related data or assessment sets to further clarify what you sense.

ASSESSMENT: EXPERTISE COMES WITH TIME AND PRACTICE

No individual nurse invented or owns nursing skills; they come with practice and experience. Often what is viewed as "normal" doesn't seem so until you have observed a condition reflecting grossly "abnormal." Discrete heart murmurs are more easily heard after you have heard a dramatic heart murmur; pupils are always evaluated singularly as well as together. You will learn to use comparisons in assessment.

Consider as you listen to the lung sounds of a patient, how does the left side sound as compared with the right side? Compare what you perceive as the "abnormal" with its opposing, symmetrical "normal." It is especially important to document "normals" in order to clearly understand any pathology. Many institutions use check lists to document such normals.

As you begin your practice, use scrap paper and write down what you see or hear so as not to miss or forget your findings. Later on, transfer your findings to the checklist. Practice your assessment *and charting* on friends or peers. Such efforts will help you become more competent in recognizing normal findings and charting them. It is helpful to repeat these skills as much as possible to achieve proficiency. Performing charting will also help you develop a rhythmic and fluid style and to more automatically include pertinent data in the order of your chosen format.

 Exercise 5.6

Match the normal documented finding with the appropriate area being assessed.

1. Lung _____
2. Heart rate _____
3. Knee reflex _____
4. Eye _____
5. Bowel sounds _____
6. Gait _____
7. Level of consciousness _____

A. Pupils equal, round, reactive to light and accommodation [PERRLA], visual acuity 20/20, ACD [anterior chamber depth] +2, IOP [intraocular pressure] 18, corneas clear

B. +2, bil (bilateral)

C. Alert and oriented [A & O] × 3 [person, place, time]

D. Normal range, × 4 quadrants

E. Fields clear bil (bilaterally), equal expansion, RR 14

F. Stable and coordinated

G. HR 72, regular, $\bar{s}$ murmur

NANDA DIAGNOSES: SUBJECTIVE AND OBJECTIVE INFORMATION

NANDA defines specific criteria a patient should meet for each nursing diagnosis. The data supporting the ND criteria can be objective, subjective, or both. Through the evaluation of the data, a nurse must demonstrate how the ND applies. In some instances subjective patient findings are the objective observations forming basis for the ND. Many psychosocial factors can be regarded as subjective information and are applied in this sense.

For instance, in determining if a patient is at risk for social isolation upon discharge, one objective criteria might be if the patient is a widow. Being a widow in itself does not necessarily constitute isolation, but it could easily be prognostic, if not diagnostic. The observation suggesting potential for social isolation needs to be supported by objective description of behaviors, such as "pt. withdrawn, avoids eye contact, does not engage in self-care" as well as patient's stated feelings. If upon further assessment and inquiry you find that the patient is demonstrating tendencies toward isolation, such supporting information would need to be added.

USING OBJECTIVE CRITERIA TO FORMULATE NURSING DIAGNOSES

There are explicit written criteria for forming each ND. The ND is considered objective if there are a minimum number of criteria applicable in an individual case. Objective and subjective values are considered in the criteria.

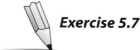

Exercise 5.7

Match the ND with the appropriate group of documented conditions.

1. Infection, risk for _____
2. Mobility impaired _____
3. Nutrition altered, less than body requirements _____
4. Coping, ineffective _____
5. Hyperthermia _____

A. Nausea, vomiting and diarrhea (N, V, D); aversion to food; dysphagia
B. Three hours post-op appendectomy, disoriented, c/o pain
C. 83 y/o, M, RR = 24, dyspnea, cough, 3 pillows for comfort
D. Neg. eye contact, wringing hands, limited responses
E. T = 102°F, flushed, diaphoretic, restless, c/o thirst

MAKING GOALS OBJECTIVE: USING OBJECTIVE PARAMETERS

Quality assurance mandates require that stated goals for patient care have measurable outcomes. If the ND refers to stress, your nursing goals may not simply be to eliminate the problem of stress for the patient. The goals also need to clearly state achievable, measurable outcomes. If your nursing goal is to decrease stress, then define what that means and by what parameters you will assess the outcome. Recording that the patient "appears calmer" has no supportive objective data and means nothing to a chart review team. Think in terms that define and measure the expected outcome.

Outcome and its subsequent evaluation should be thought of as inseparable. Even if the outcome you select does not have the predicted or anticipated results, it still needs to be able to be assessed and recorded as to its measured effect. Not all patients will recover; wellness and normalcy will not be restored in every patient. As a nurse, you do not "get into trouble" because the patient does not regain full functioning. Your job, however, is to assess and reassess your patients for what is needed from a nursing perspective. You plan, implement, and evaluate the effectiveness of your care.

DEALING WITH OBNOXIOUS PATIENTS

Patients are not usually in a hospital or clinic because they feel well, and they are not always in good moods. It is easier for people to be pleasant and more social when they feel good rather than a person who is ill or injured. Many times, patients can be obnoxious and uncooperative. It is irrelevant whether this is a reflection of actual personality or a manifestation of how they feel. Your notes should not reflect subjective comments about the patient's effect on you or the staff.

Choose descriptors about a patient very carefully. If the patient has a potential to be harmful to self and others, record the actions that make this an actual, true observation. If a patient refuses to cooperate with care requests, write only about actions that support the assertion and your interventions in teaching the patient why a particular medicine or procedure is indicated.

Patients are allowed to choose their care or the type of care they permit. This is more commonly known as "The Patient's Bill of Rights" and one of a nurse's strongest professional charges is to advocate for the patient according to his or her rights. Chapter 8 will cover your nursing responsibilities to the patient's rights in more detail. For now, however, consider the impact of your written record. It may be far less judgmental to note that a patient has chosen to "decline" care than to use a trigger word like "refused." Similarly, terms such as "noncompliant," "belligerent," or "hostile" when discussing whether a patient is cooperative or not are generally to be avoided due to their potential for judgmental value.

HEALTH CARE IS PERSONAL TO THE PATIENT

Patients do take their care and interactions with staff personally. It is their health and care that is being planned and implemented. Patients may feel that they have no control over their own body or the disease that is affecting their usual state of wellness. Or, a patient may feel overwhelmed by the lack of familiarity with their surroundings and events.

A patient's behavior or state of comfort may reflect a need for control (NANDA dx). The words used by caregivers in front of the patient or family members are vital. Use simple language to explain care and procedures. Individualize your interviewing to reflect a patient's ability to understand. Literacy, education, and culture must be considered. Do remember in all cases that the language health care professionals use is not always familiar to the patient. Their experience may be from watching TV and movies or from experiential input from past situations by themselves, family, and neighbors.

MAKING NOTES MORE OBJECTIVE: AVOID PERSONALIZATION

Refer back to Exercise 2.4. There is no effective way to note tone of voice or inflection in charting. What you document will be interpreted by the reader based on his or her own biases and information.

Health care staff, quality assurance people, or legal reviewers do not know or care if you may have had a bad day or poor rapport with a patient. Avoid any written reaction to patient behavior.

Documenting your judgment-based information accurately is a difficult task to learn. This workbook has been describing some of the more common instances you might assess or chart in a less than objective manner. It takes time to learn to discriminate, and some practicing nurses may not be good role models.

 Exercise 5.8

Match each personalized word with its more objective description.

1. Fat _____
2. Gross _____
3. Overwhelmed _____
4. Hostile _____
5. Stinks _____
6. Drunk _____
7. Sad _____
8. Refusing _____
9. Mean _____
10. Behaving badly _____

A. Chooses not to comply with staff verbal requests
B. Demonstrating angry behaviors
C. ETOH noted as smell on breath
D. Less than controlled
E. Malodorous
F. Purposeful, aggressive actions directed at staff
G. Purposeful statements, expressing emotion, directed at staff
H. Obese
I. Objectionable
J. Withdrawn, not making eye contact, shortened answers to questions

INTUITIVE DATA: THE "HUNCH" FACTOR

How does a dog hear sounds that humans cannot? How does a smaller animal sense danger of a nearby predator? How can "an impending sense of doom" be assessed as an adverse effect of a new medication taken by a patient? If a nurse walks into a patient's room a senses that something is wrong, is that simply an indiscriminate feeling on the part of the nurse or is the nurse employing more cultivated assessment capabilities?

BOX 5.5

Degrees of Description

This list of similar descriptive words demonstrates varied degrees of emphasis that language can communicate. The difference may be slight but very meaningful.

Color vs. Inflammation

Documenting the color of skin or wound does not define a diagnosis. Documenting "inflammation" states a physiologic process that is associated with a change in color.

Diaphoresis vs. Clammy

Clammy and diaphoretic are not synonyms but are often wrongly used interchangeably.

Temperature vs. Fever

Everyone has a temperature; fever refers to a temperature that is higher than normal.

Alert vs. Obtunded

This demonstrates an antonym relationship of subjective extremes. An alert person may become confused or demonstrate some confusion; it is not likely that an obtunded patient could be assessed for orientation.

In response, consider how we know it is windy; how we "see" the wind? One might feel wind or observe evidence of wind in the atmosphere, but one cannot actually see wind with the naked eye.

The hunch a nurse uses to sense something is or is not right with a patient may actually be based in refined abilities of perceptiveness and observation in combination with experience and practice. Experienced nurses recognize and incorporate these subtle and often nearly imperceptible values into their patient's assessment.

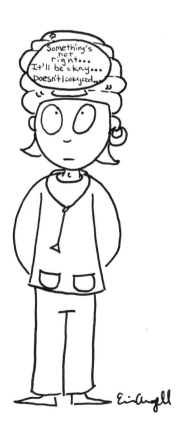

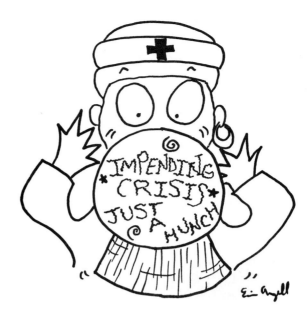

Little clues often lead to questions or further assessments, which promote subjective statements from the patients to support the nurse's assertion, the nurse's hunch.

Angina is a medical diagnosis, yet like the wind a physician cannot completely measure or "see" angina. The physician has to relate the patient's complaint with laboratory analyses and electrocardiograms to confirm the lack of pathological evidence of heart muscle damage in conjunction with the patient's stated symptoms. However, angina pain felt by a patient is in fact very real and may often be a preliminary sign of impending heart damage or attack.

An experienced practitioner does not disregard complaints without follow-up investigation. If a patient in a critical situation tells a nurse, "I am going to die," it sends chills up the spine of the nurse because most often, it is true. Do not ignore what a patient may say; do not disregard what your hunch is telling you. It is frequently an extremely important clue about a patient's status and should not be taken lightly or frivolously. Expert practitioners do not always understand the origin of a hunch but they most often respond with watchfulness for the potential problem that lingers in the extreme periphery.

It is important that guesses or hunches not be ignored and should be explored further. Actual assessment data often support the intuitive suspicion affecting patient outcome.

Deciding how to discuss "gut" feelings or the sense that a patient is "going south" in the absence of supporting objective data is one of the most difficult problems in nursing. It does not belong in the chart. And often providers are not interested in the nurse's feelings even if based on extensive past experience.

Passing data through verbal report and the judicious use of nursing diagnoses or prevention plans based on "potential for" information alerts other staff to be watchful for symptoms that may corroborate your suspicion.

SUMMARY

As you make more objective, professional notations in the patient record, you will notice that your systems for assessment and moving within the subjective world of the patient will begin to standardize. You will notice that as you achieve objectivity you develop consistency. This is your goal, this is what you will work toward during your professional career. The way we document often reflects the manner in which we practice. It is not only a medical necessity that nurses learn to discriminate between the subjective and the objective patient information, but it is also a legal and financial imperative that nurses document the difference.

Answer Guide

Exercise 5.1

1. character
   Common: traits that define a person's integrity or behavior; a shorthand symbol that represents a value of some description; slang that portrays behavior as interesting and singular
   Technical: traits that describe in detail a specific complaint or symptom

2. decline
   Common: refuse; reject; descend
   Technical: refuse; to deteriorate in condition

3. refuse
   Common: declined to accept or allow; discard as worthless
   Technical: declined to do or allow

4. failure
   Common: to fall short or be deficient; unsuccessful
   Technical: inability to function; to miss medical appointment

5. radiation
   Common: emitting rays; glowing manifestation
   Technical: to spread from a focal area

6. irreversible
   Common: impossible to reverse
   Technical: condition that cannot be turned back

7. incompetence
   Common: not qualified
   Technical: organs that are not functioning properly; person legally proclaimed unable to manage his or her own affairs

8. compliant
   Common: yielding
   Technical: measure by which an organ deforms or distends; adheres to recommended course of treatment

9. ordinary
   Common: usual; not exceptional
   Technical: within a standard, expected performance standard

10. complaint
    Common: expressed dissatisfaction; formal legal charge by plaintiff
    Technical: ailment, problem, or symptom expressed by patient

11. deviant
    Common: abandoning normal or proscribed behavior; different from normal; abnormal, sometimes criminal, behavior
    Technical: reaction that fails to respond in expected fashion; differing from standard or norm

12. bias
    Common: diagonal line across grain of fabric; preference that interferes with impartial judgment
    Technical: prejudiced or subjective attitude; not objectively represented in a balanced fashion

13. objective
Common: material rather than mental concept; uninfluenced by personal feelings
Technical: clinical sign that can be seen heard or measured; goal; lens of microscope

14. subjective
Common: personal
Technical: symptom, sensation, or assessment that cannot be measured or observed

15. cretin
Common: dolt or idiot
Technical: individual with stunted physical growth or mental ability

16. expel
Common: dismiss, drive out
Technical: emit gas or matter from a body cavity

17. discipline
Common: punishment; training for strict order or behavior
Technical: specific medical specialty

18. indolent
Common: lazy
Technical: not active, not an active medical problem

19. insipid
Common: dull; without flavor or tasteless
Technical: not arousing interest; vague

20. noncompliant
Common: not malleable
Technical: not able or willing to comply with treatment regimen

21. obese
Common: extremely overweight
Technical: abnormally overweight by a defined percentage

22. vapid
Common: not interested; not lively
Technical: dull; listless

Exercise 5.2

1. whining—complaint
2. smells bad—poor hygiene
3. denies—states no
4. refuse—decline
5. difficult—uncooperative to verbal request
6. stutter—hesitant speech
7. asleep—resting with eyes closed
8. drunk—smell of alcohol noted on breath
9. noncompliant—unable to complete staff requests
10. homeless—states no permanent residence
11. fussy—noted to be crying at intervals
12. possible CVA—witnessed loss of motor functions unilaterally

Exercise 5.3

1. C;   2. F;   3. H;   4. D;   5. G;   6. E;   7. B;   8. I;   9. A

Exercise 5.4

1. poor hygiene—foul smelling odor, hair matted, unkempt appearance, shoes worn without socks
2. bad stutter—language pattern reflecting repetitive speech habits and difficulty with pronunciation of certain words
3. disease—evidence of pathological process affecting state of wellness
4. old—age stated in years
5. cultural bias—potential expressed for a predetermined opinion relating to one's cultural orientation
6. race—ethnicity
7. class—subjectively based determination of one's financial, social, or economical status
8. morals—ethical or religious opinion, judgment, determination, or value
9. religious—statement indicating someone's declared orientation to religious preference or that someone espouses theologically based values
10. educational level—statement indicating an individual's degree or level of formal education

Exercise 5.5

1. tumor
2. growth
3. malignancy, inoperable cancer
4. denied, alcoholic, drunk
5. uncooperative, refused
6. minor
7. abusive, belligerent, noncompliant
8. homeless, terrible, illiterate
9. bizarre, demented
10. disabled

Exercise 5.6

1. E;   2. G;   3. B;   4. A;   5. D;   6. F;   7. C

Exercise 5.7

1. C;   2. B;   3. A;   4. D;   5. E

Exercise 5.8

1. H;   2. I;   3. D;   4. B;   5. E;   6. C;   7. J;   8. A;   9. F;   10. G

CHAPTER 6

Follow-Up Questions for the Beginner

WORD LIST

persistent	rebound	exquisite
advanced	excursion	local
vegetative	dilate	quadrant
reversible	injection	ribbon
mass	boring	loose
anterior	pounding	
murmur	thready	

 Exercise 6.1

Each item in the word list has both common and technical meanings. Match each word with its corresponding set of definitions and compare the intent or usage of the terms as both common and technical words.

1. _____
   Common: person from a particular area; branch of labor union
   Technical: not general or systemic; anesthetic limited to one area

2. _____
   Common: elaborately done; beautiful
   Technical: intense, keen, sharp

3. _____
   Common: enduring; continuing firmly in spite of obstacle
   Technical: obstinate continuation, despite the environmental conditions

4. _____
   Common: highly developed; complex
   Technical: far along in course

5. _____
   Common: relating to plants or plant growth; capable of growth
   Technical: not active; growing or functioning involuntarily or unconsciously

6. _____
   Common: turned backward in position, order, or direction
   Technical: turning in opposite direction of disease, symptom, or state

7. _____
   Common: not tightly fastened, bound, stapled, or bundled; not exact in interpretation; demonstrating lack of restraint; immoral
   Technical: not formed or bound together in reference to stool or tissue; mental associations implying disordered thought process

8. _____
   Common: low continuous sound; mutter
   Technical: soft sound heard while listening to heart or vessels

9. _____
   Common: forcing one element (gas or liquid) into another (ground); introducing a subject into a discussion
   Technical: introducing medicine into tissue or vein; congestion or hyperemia, as with a red eye

10. _____
    Common: dull; repetitive
    Technical: drilling or digging sensation

11. _____
    Common: striking repeatedly; crushing by forceful beating
    Technical: heavy throbbing sensation

12. _____
    Common: having to do with fibrous strands twisted together; ridges on screws or bolts; common element that is cohesive
    Technical: description of pulse quality that is weaker and fairly rapid, often indicating hypovolemia

13. _____
    Common: short trip or outing usually for pleasure; digression
    Technical: deviation from expected normal course

14. _____
    Common: altitude determining instrument; mathematical plane
    Technical: division of an anatomical region for purpose of description

15. _____
    Common: nonspecific quantity or amount of matter; reference to greatest number of members of common group; religious celebration
    Technical: number of cells grouped together, such as tumor; physical properties of matter that give it measurable dimensions

16. _____
    Common: bounce or spring back; recover after a let down
    Technical: sudden contraction of muscle after relaxation; sudden response to an activity or treatment after the stimulus has been removed

17. _____
    Common: enlarge or expand
    Technical: enlarge cavity either through intention, disease process, or normal response

18. _____
    Common: front location
    Technical: reference in anatomical position to areas facing forward

19. _____
    Common: narrow strip of cloth or decorative fabric
    Technical: stool formed flat and narrow

GATHERING DATA

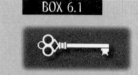

General medical-surgical nursing books as well as texts devoted to assessment skills should be your primary sources for how-to and hands-on physical assessment. The case studies here will focus on appropriate questions that are instrumental in eliciting specific information from the patient relating to symptom descriptors: location, quality, quantity, chronology, setting, associated manifestations, alleviating and aggravating factors, and meaning to the patient.

Case Study 6.1a

Symptom Interview: Chief Complaint

Mr. X is admitted to your unit with a chief complaint of abdominal pain, Left Lower Quadrant (LLQ). He is lying in a supine position with the side rails raised when you enter the room responding to his call signal. You have hardly reached his bedside when Mr. X says, "Nurse, can you do something about this pain?" To which you reply, "Where are you having pain?"

BOX 6.1

Symptom Descriptors

Location

Anterior, posterior, aspect, upper, outer, quadrants, inner, midline, symmetry, supine, prone, clock use, measurements, mid, left, right, proximal, distal, sub-, generalized, local, deep shallow

Quality

Objective parameters, 1–10, facies pain scale, symbols, mild, moderate, severe, exquisite, profuse, radiating, ROM, degrees of motion, bounding, pounding, thready, sharp, dull, "the worst HA ever," rapid, boring

Quantity

Persistent, intermittent, per hour, constant, per week, numeration, regular, irregular, profuse, prolific, relentless, occasional, weekly, hourly, monthly, quarterly, yearly

Chronology

Onset, duration, pattern of symptom, increase, decrease, timing, direct relation to series of events related to outcome, timing of bruises, event relationship, seasonal, relationship to mealtime, post fasting, time of day, monthly, sudden, insidious

Setting

Position (may affect location), timing, meals, p, q, exposure at home or work, activity level, who or what present

Associated Manifestations

What, where, always, subjective observation, direct quote, coincidence, precursor, related/unrelated symptom observations, comorbid factors, covert, occult, overt

Alleviating/Aggravating Factors

Worse, better, increased, decreased, position, treatment, medication, stress, objective or subjective outcomes, outcome measurement tools, alternative medicine, meditation, prayer, weather, increase/decrease activity, pillow count, positioning, OTC or home remedies

Meaning to Patient

Subjective, direct quote, objective, denial, changes, work, self-esteem, lifestyle interruption, economic impact, insurance, disruption of routine

---

BOX 6.2

General Appearance

By documenting the general appearance of a patient, you are describing your impression of the patient's look, demeanor, and well-being when presenting for care. This first, and often underestimated, category in the review of systems (ROS) provides a baseline by which you will measure the patient's progress as he or she receives care. It is more complex than "looks good" or "looks bad" and should convey the intended impression. In simple terms, how sick, or well, does the patient appear to be prior to receiving care for this visit?

You may also notice "wasting" and "puffy" appearance. While constitutional symptoms such as nausea, vomiting, diarrhea, and appetite dysfunction are not always visually observable, the effects of these symptoms may be obvious to an experienced eye.

The danger of recording that a patient does not "look" sick lies in the effect the statement may have on other caregivers, or yourself, taking the patient's complaints seriously. Avoid judging the patient's veracity, or intentions, when describing the problem. Insidious and occult problems may be even further masked by your interpretation of

how the patient might be "expected" to appear under a given set of conditions as opposed to how he or she actually appears.

Appearance can often be altered by a person's ethnicity and by their cultural or learned response to a given condition. How the patient feels about themselves may depend upon displaying no outward weakness, on being "brave" or "stoic." The patient may consider even the most life-threatening conditions as signs of weakness. Some personalities function only when in complete control of all situations, potentially misleading your "impression" of the patient.

Legally you must record the patient's appearance as you perceive it. Your charting may have consequences for care that you cannot predict. Therefore, it is highly recommended that you support your subjective impression with observable physical data. For instance, if a patient presents with severe pain but demonstrates no associated characteristics, record this. Observe the patient closely; jaw tightening, clenched fists or teeth, or other subtle indicators that may otherwise be overlooked.

The first question you asked focuses on the location of the pain expressed by your patient. While it seems obvious that pain is Mr. X's chief complaint, it is dangerous to assume that any complaint is *necessarily* related to a patient's admitting problem, particularly in patients with multisystem involvement or concurrent diagnosis. Note that the word *necessarily* does not mean possible or probable; it refers to situations in which conditions are certain to occur. Anticipated outcomes or responses may not transpire, and patients respond contrary to expectations. Don't assume anything.

Thorough investigation will yield complete and specific information related to your patient's complaints and associated symptoms. It is important to understand that patients seek health care when they are sick. Even with health care moving toward the health promotion model, health care continues to be primarily secondary and tertiary care. You will often be exploring health problems. If you are working in an acute care or skilled nursing setting you will be seeing patients who are sick enough to require acute institutional care. The questions you ask will guide your patients to be precise in their symptom descriptions without being led to agree to information that may not be correct.

It is helpful to memorize the characteristics of a symptom (or carry a list to cue your memory) and to follow a routine pattern of questioning. This will help you to avoid omitting vital information. Eventually you will establish a pattern of interviewing that will yield a precise data base for each patient and will establish guidelines for providing individualized and problem-specific nursing care.

SYMPTOM CHARACTERISTICS

The review of systems (ROS) format is used throughout this chapter to provide the tools necessary to gather data. Moving from broad-based questions to the very precise, these questions can usually be generalized; that is, they can be adapted for and applicable to many different patient situations.

Each body system must be considered for external features as well as for the complete three-dimensional aspect. This will become clearer as you review each of the systems for its particular characteristics. As you progress through the chapter, you may become aware of the consistent and repetitive data collection process. As with nursing process it is imperative to learn the concepts related to correct documentation of data from the ROS. If you have a routine for observing and collecting information and know the words to use to record it, you will see that it clearly becomes a matter of repetition and application.

LOCATION

The location of a given symptom should be isolated as specifically as possible so that caregivers can offer appropriate treatment. Nurses have the opportunity for a closer, more personal relationship with the patient than the medical provider and are more likely to elicit concise and helpful information. Even with the time constraints on nursing care of the hospitalized patient, nurses who can make

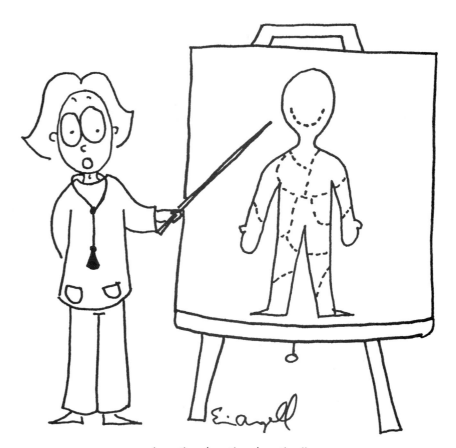

Location, location, location!!

BOX 6.3

Descriptors ROS

General—weight (weight $\Delta \uparrow\downarrow$), appetite, weakness, fever, fatigue

Skin—Δ hair or nails, dermatologic rashes or lesions, moisture, color, flaking, pruritis, bumps, infestations (treatment for infestation), exposures to toxins (work, household, incidental)

Head—pain, hx of injury

Eyes—visual acuity, $\Delta \uparrow\downarrow$, glasses, contacts, IOL [intraocular lens], pain, drainage, excess watering, conjunctival redness, visual disturbance, family history

Ears—hearing, pain, infection hx, dizziness, cerumen, drainage

Nose, Sinus—congestion, drainage, nosebleeds, infection (colds, sinus)

Mouth, Throat—dental hx (caries, dentures, hygiene, checkups), bleeding, lesions, taste, vocal Δ (hoarseness, laryngitis), mouth hydration

Neck—pain, lumps, swelling, ROM (full/limited, stiffness)

Breasts—symmetry, pain, lumps, nipple discharge, BSE

Respiratory—rate, tone, pitch, excursion, wheezing, cough, hemoptysis, sputum production, TB exposure, sleep interruption and position of rest (number of pillows)

Cardiac—HR, regular, BP, murmur, pain, arrhythmias, family hx

Gastrointestinal—digestive problems (heartburn, swallowing, food intolerance), nausea, vomiting, diarrhea, constipation, abdominal pain, bowel sounds, belching, passing gas, Δ in stool (consistency, size, color)

Urinary—frequency, itching, burning, hesitancy, color, odor, concentration, output (related to intake), force of stream, hematuria

Peripheral Vascular—pain, cramping, color, warmth, lesions, hair growth

Musculoskeletal—pain, stiffness, weakness, Δ mobility or ROM, tenderness

Neurologic—numbness, tingling, weakness, gait Δ, seizures, fainting, tremors

Hematologic—bleeding, fatigue, bruising

Endocrine—polyphagia, polyuria, polydipsia, heat/cold intolerance, weight Δ

Psychiatric—mood variations, crying, hysteria, hx of depression

Genital—

Male—swelling/masses, pain, penile discharge, TSE, sexual function, STD hx

Female—onset of menarche, P, G, TAB, SAB (para, gravida, therapeutic abortion, spontaneous abortion), regularity, frequency, flow, duration, LNMP [last normal menstrual period], discharge, nonmenstrual bleeding, lumps, infection, itching, sexual function, STD hx, menopause, DES (diethylstilbestrol)

BOX 6.4

Location

The skin is the body's largest organ system and provides a protective covering for the rest of the body systems. Use the other body systems as landmarks when it is necessary to describe the location of a skin-related symptom. Common disorders related to (r/t) the skin and which have symptoms that require precise description are pruritis (itch), lesions, pain, burning, rashes, wounds, and circulatory dysfunction. Landmarks that will help you describe the broad location of such disorders on the skin are the musculoskeletal system, joints, symmetrical orientations or specific organ location. You may want to review Exercise 6.3 with its anatomical reference points.

Hair and nails are included in this system and may or may not need separate description. A patient who has normal head and body hair needs little reference after the admitting history and physical (H & P), although location of primary hair loss related to disease or treatment should be noted. The patient who presents with thinning, breakable hair or evidence of rapid loss may need further description of such deficits.

Nails and nailbeds can be indicators of disease process. Location of nails is not usually an issue, with the exception of an absent nail.

(continued on next page)

BOX 6.4—*Continued*

Finding a location of a skin symptom can be as easy as asking a patient to point to the spot that is affected. Certainly sight and touch are ways to determine exact locations. The skin, unless hidden under the dressings of a nonverbal patient, provides visual clues. It is your job to describe the location of a disorder and to provide a verbal picture that recalls the specific description to any member of the health care team. Musculoskeletal landmarks help define broad locations on the skin along with specific organ locations and anatomical positioning related to extremities.

The external physical exam includes description of location or placement of any affected system. For example, an eye exam should include an overview and description of the general appearance of the eyes. Use your visual observation skills to look at your patient and see if the eyes are placed symmetrically and if the external features are equal. While a person's left and right sides are not exact mirror images there should be no remarkable deviations. (Imagine seeing someone who has one normal eye and the other swollen shut and discolored in a fight.) Use the visual external exam to look for deviations from what we expect from a *normal* exam. You will compare the left eye to the right, in effect, using the patient as their own reference point and control. Then describe what you see.

Internal *ocular* (r/t the eye) symptoms, felt and described by the patient present a greater documentation challenge. For instance the patient reports "eye pain." You will determine if the pain is located external to the ocular *globe, upper or lower lid, or surrounding bone (orbit) and tissue.* Headache pain is often referred to as eye pain when it is located posterior to the eyeball. Since each eye is essentially round, clock locations are often used to describe the location of a stated complaint. For instance you can document: soft tissue mass, corneal border, 5 o'clock (common description for a pterygium).

Descriptors common to these systems are derived from anatomical landmarks and conditions that may affect these systems. However we often see medical terms used that have more common reference in other body systems. For example "nasolabial fold" describes the portion of the nose that approximates the upper lip. Most people think of the word labia in relation to female genitalia. *Labia*, however, refer to *lips;* the root of the word and its actual definition are vital to our understanding.

External exam of the thorax and abdomen uses the same visual skills as noted here. You record symmetry of the breasts, comparing one side to the other, noting the position on the body. A symptom evident on one side can be compared with the absence of the symptom on the other. For instance, a small breast mass may be located in the left lower breast quadrant, at 0700. The opposing side may be smooth and soft or be cystic, but can be used for comparison. Breast tissue and type may also be described and should be relatively symmetrical side to side. Look for obvious markings and for scars from any prior wound or surgery.

To evaluate the location of symptoms near the internal organs you usually rely on assessment skills that allow you to estimate the position. Auscultation and palpation allow you to establish a more exact position of internal organs. With lungs and other respiratory organs as well as the heart and vascular system, you can use your stethoscope to listen and locate normal or abnormal findings. You can compare the actual findings to the expected values. Anatomical location is estimated as closely as possible in order for you to assess the problem, to plan an appropriate intervention, and in order to evaluate the outcome of care. You likely will not be the nurse to a specific patient for the duration of his or her complaint. Other caregivers must be able to read your description and assess the area at the location you described.

time for building a more therapeutic relationship will usually assist the patient more effectively.

One of the most common symptoms you will explore is pain. The examples presented here will focus on pain in relation to the categories in the ROS. The exercises may also include additional symptom descriptors with which you will be able to supplement your knowledge throughout the chapter.

Exercise 6.2

The words below are used to anatomically place a symptom. Write definitions for the following terms, looking up those that are unfamiliar to you in your medical dictionary.

1. unilateral _____
2. bilateral _____
3. anterior _____
4. posterior _____
5. aspect _____
6. upper _____
7. outer _____
8. quadrants _____
9. inner _____
10. midline _____
11. symmetry _____
12. supine _____
13. prone _____
14. measurement _____
15. mid- _____
16. left _____
17. right _____
18. proximal _____
19. distal _____
20. sub- _____

As you observe the patient's normal and symmetrical features, are you noticing a pattern? Think of the ways in which nurses are taught to compare and contrast. Observing pupils, gait, grip strength, sensory deficits, even facial droops are all examples of ways nurses are taught to consider the patient's own body systems and functions to establish a basis of comparison. Examples of descriptive words are *symmetry, equality, midline, equidistant.* A comparative analysis might state that a "palpable mass is located at the rt nasolabial fold with no evidence of a mass on the lt." Generally speaking, if there is a positive finding on one side; that is, your assessment reveals findings that are not necessarily considered within normal limits, then that observation is noted with an exact, anatomically specific description. The symmetrical, anatomical opposite side of any finding may serve as a control against which data, measurements, or observations can be compared.

Exercise 6.3

Label Figure 6.1 with the applicable location descriptors. If you use a prefix be sure to add the correct word that completes the anatomical description, for instance, substernal or intercostal.

anterior patellar

axillary

distal femoral

midclavicular

midepigastric

midsternal

periorbital

submandibular

suprapubic

umbilical

Figure 6.1

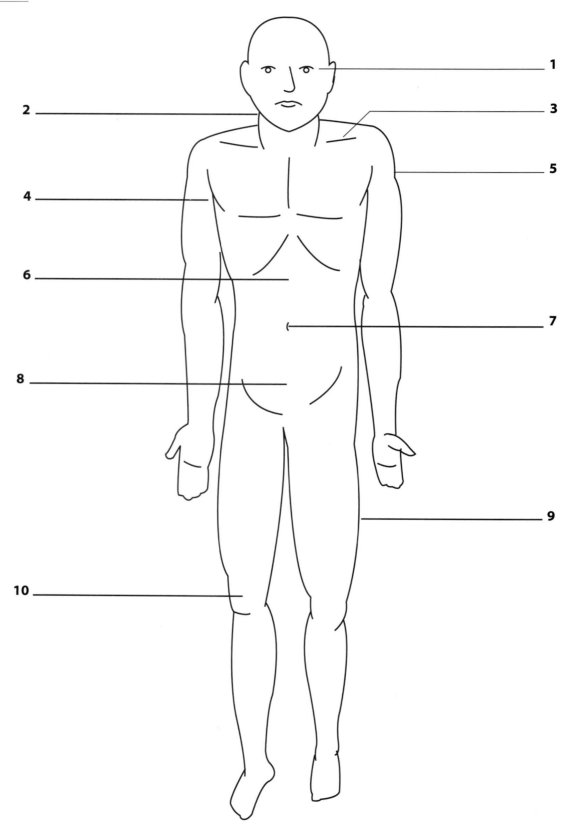

The location of visual findings can be quantitatively measured and very exact. In certain cases, such as when noting or documenting traumatic injuries, photographs may be used with a measuring apparatus in place to determine or compare scale.

Describing the precise location of subjective symptoms is far more difficult. In this instance, you are relying on the patient's comprehension and language ability. With an unconscious patient, a child, or a non-English-speaking patient, your own assessment and communication skills are critical in narrowing the description to reflect an accurate and clear representation of a given circumstance.

You are learning words associated with the location of symptoms in the individual systems. Choose the words that most succinctly pinpoint the location of a described normal finding or patient complaint. Remember that as you become an expert on the variations of normal findings you will also be learning to recognize abnormal findings.

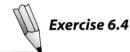

Exercise 6.4

When interviewing the patient about location, choose the *better* follow-up question in the following scenarios:

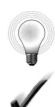

Example:

Mr. X says that the pain is in his "gut." You:
a. Ask him to point to the spot where the pain is most noticeable.
b. Ask what he means by gut.
c. Ask if it is greater on the left than right side.

Answer "a."

1. Mr. Y states his back is itching and burning. You ask:
   a. What do you mean when you say "back"?
   b. Where exactly on your back is the itching and burning located?
   c. Does it itch more than it burns?

2. A woman arrived holding her head stating, "I can't take it anymore." You ask:
   a. Why didn't you take some medication?
   b. What can't you take anymore?
   c. Is there a pain somewhere in your head?

3. The child pointed to his arm and said it felt "funny." You ask:
   a. Does it feel funnier than yesterday?
   b. Show me with your finger the spot that feels funny.
   c. Did it begin on the playground at school today?

4. Miss Y. was lying absolutely still, with hands clenched at her side. You ask:
   a. Is there someplace on your body that is causing you discomfort right now?
   b. Are you nervous about anything?
   c. Is there something I can help you with?

5. Mr. Z was carried in by his family who said he was having an "attack." You ask:
   a. When did this start?
   b. Did he say anything was wrong before he stopped talking?
   c. Do you have any sense or idea of where it's hurting him?

QUALITY

The quality of a given symptom as expressed verbally by the patient is the primary measurement of the degree of impact the symptom has on the patient. It is one of the most profound descriptors. It is vital in the evaluation of a symptom, yet because of its inherently subjective nature, it is perhaps the most difficult for a caregiver to quantify.

As you investigate the quality of a symptom you will be asking your patient to use words or indicate according to a scale the measure and character of their own reaction to that specific symptom. The parameters the nurse uses are quantifiable only against the patient's own historical reference to like events from his or her past. When suggesting possible ways to quantify the degree or quality of the symptom that the patient is experiencing, the nurse adds a potential for a degree of bias. While it is true that the patient chooses how best to describe the symptom in question, the process of questioning in order to determine the quality is ripe for bias.

Case Study 6.1b
Charting example: Mr. X
1400: c/o "dull, burning" pain, LLQ (abd).
Verbal report
1400: c/o pain LLQ, Δ from sharp to dull & burning.

As the patient describes the quality of the symptom, you will also be comparing and evaluating the patient's perception of that symptom against what would usually be expected in similar circumstances for other patients. You might inadvertently be responsible for any further biases in recording the patient's complaint if you compare and then question the patient's reliability against what you usually expect from a particular finding. In actuality, while you may question if the patient complaint is consistent with what is routinely expected,

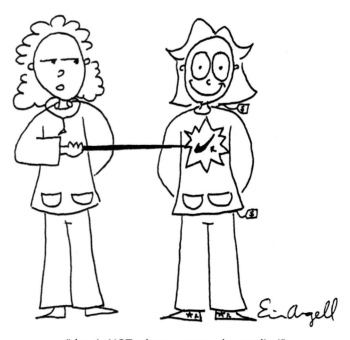

"that is NOT what we mean by quality!"

you need to be very cautious not to subjectively determine a patient symptom inconsistent.

When learning to quantify a patient's subjective parameters, nurses should use terminology that they *always* apply to a specific, similarly reported complaint. For instance there are many words to describe pain; sharp, dull, throbbing, boring, or cutting. If you frequently use a pain scale methodology and combine numerical values obtained from the scales with the more common verbal pain descriptors, you will know with consistency and accuracy what you intended if you noted "moderate pain."

If the symptom you are describing can be observed, such as drainage or expectoration, you are able to quantify character, color, consistency, amount, and viscosity in order to most correctly record the nature and quality of the drainage fluid.

BOX 6.5

Quality of a Symptom

Language that describes quality emphasizes how the symptom feels, how it seems, or what it "acts" like to the patient. "Quality" descriptors are words the patient would use to describe what the symptom feels like. It also characterizes the nature of the symptom. The quality differs from quantity, but is best expressed in measurable or quantifiable terms. "Pain" is an easy reference in learning to describe quality, but a very difficult and precise symptom for you to learn to describe, because no one but the patient feels and therefore describes the pain exactly the same way.

Read the following list of descriptors that are frequently used to describe these symptoms:

Pain: mild, moderate, severe, exquisite, sharp, dull, boring, burning, searing, pressure, grabbing, pulsing, radiating, occult

Pulse Quality: strong, bounding, weak, thready, labile, regular, irregular

Respirations: regular, agonal, shallow, deep

Constitutional Symptoms: fatigue, malaise, weary, impending doom, achy, weak

The quality of any symptom is based on the subjective perception of that symptom by the patient. The patient's quoted words can be most effective. To quantify the description, consider asking the patient to use a common reference scale tool.

The effects of the quality of a stated problem on a patient can also be observed by you. You have many objectively based, quantifiable tools to support your subjectively determined parameter. Consider the intoxicated patient. A layperson may simply state that the person is "drunk." You may ask

the patient if they have consumed any alcohol as you observe the patient for slurred speech, unsteady gait, blurry eyes, nystagmus, or smell of alcohol on the breath. Evidence of these findings may physically support your determination that a person is intoxicated or certainly under the effects of alcohol in their system.

Read the following modifiers used to describe these physical signs:

Bruises: ecchymotic, color scale (red, blue, black, green, yellow), faded, raised, measurement (in mm)

Lacerations: depth (superficial, submucosal, deep sub-q, extending to . . .), anatomical placement, scale of degrees (1–5°)

Constitutional: pale, diaphoretic, flushed, obtunded, moribund, cachectic, obese

The quality of a patient's consciousness and/or demeanor is measured by the Glasgow coma scale, by the degree of alertness as measured by orientation to time, place, and person, as well as by tools such as the Mini Mental Status exam. Words commonly used are: alert & oriented (A & O) × 3 (person, time, place) or number that applies, restless, combative, cooperative, appropriate, inappropriate, responsive (with measurement used, e.g., to voice, pain)

You may need to describe a lump or lesion: soft, hard, freely moving, fixed, ± pain, regular/irregular border, raise, flat, color, hairy, smooth, dry, bleeding, draining, oozing, odor.

All qualities need careful description in your note.

Exercise 6.5

Match the descriptor with its definition:

absent
accommodation
bilaterally
dry
equal
intact
light
reactive
round
warm

1. associated to two parts
2. present and in an unimpaired condition
3. not present, infers a lack of presence or finding
4. quantifies comparatively with another of similar character
5. appears to the eye to be in a circular state or condition
6. responsive to an applied stimulus
7. refers to an external source of illumination or infers a lesser state of coma or anesthesia
8. infers a sensation, feeling or presence of heat or temperature
9. infers a feeling or presence of waterless sensation or state
10. contraction or adjustment of ciliary muscles which results in circular largeness or smallness of the pupil of the eye

Exercise 6.6

Fill in the blanks with the descriptors from Exercise 6.5.

1. Pupils are _____, _____, and _____ to _____ and _____.
2. Dressing is _____.
3. Skin is _____ and _____.
4. Pedal pulse is palpable _____.
5. Reflex is _____ left lower extremity (LLE).

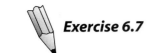

Exercise 6.7

Pick a descriptor that might be used to modify the following symptoms.

Example:

Mr. X says the L abdominal pain is different from when admitted. It had been sharp and sudden at onset but is now _____ and _____.
(dull and burning)

apex	pressure
cool	rapid
dusky	redness
exquisite	ringing
full	sensitive
granulation	serosanguineous
labored	sharp
multiple	stabbing
numbness	swelling
pale	tingling

1. Patient c/o _____ pain OS and is _____ to bright light.
2. Pt. hears _____ in ears.
3. The drainage is _____ with _____ blood clots in the tubing.
4. The healing ulcer showed _____ with no _____ or _____.
5. The heart rate was _____ and pounding, visible at the _____ on inspection of the chest.
6. Respirations were _____ and the patient's lips were _____ post expiration.
7. Abdomen felt _____ with downward _____ sensation on the bladder.
8. _____ and _____ in the L lower extremity.
9. Skin was _____ and _____
10. _____ _____ pain on palpation of LLQ of abdomen.

The addition of information regarding the change in the nature of the pain in the verbal report allows the provider or incoming staff immediate access to the information without having to review the chart to compare with previous symptom description. The change may also be noted in the written documentation but is not usually or necessarily included unless significant or definitive. Otherwise, any change, even small or transient, invites cumbersome charting prone to error.

QUANTITY

When determining the symptom characteristic of quantity, you again find patients offering vague and subjective descriptions of a symptom. You will often need to "suggest" parameters for the patient to choose from. A prime example is trying to determine if a symptom is continuous or intermittent. If the patient

BOX 6.6

Quantity

Quantity is not as clear as it seems. Measuring a subjective complaint is challenging, because you may need to explain to a patient who is not familiar with the more common measurement tools nurses employ to determine the quantity of a symptom to a patient. For instance, if a patient states that he is feeling sad, you will want more information to know if he is at risk for depression. The usual means to quantify feelings of sadness are behavioral changes in appetite, sleep habits, and sexual desire.

The behavioral changes overlap with how the symptom affects the patient's life, with what it means to the patient. Clearly as you explore a problem you will be listening to the answer in the context of the patient's overall experience and outward appearances.

If the patient is alert and able to cooperate, it is easier to quantify pain because there are fairly standard scales that can be used for comparison. You may ask a patient "On a scale of 1–10, with 10 being the worst pain you can imagine, how would you rate this pain?" You might ask a child if the pain hurts "a little, medium, or a lot" or use the Wong-Baker facies pain scale, which quantifies the look on a child's face with a numeric level of distress. Both the scale as well as the patient's base for comparison allow you assess pain with objective standards.

If, however, the patient is preverbal, demented, or aphasic, it may be much more difficult to obtain "how much" pain or experience with the presenting symptom the patient is actually experiencing.

Many observations can be measured objectively: amount of drainage, character of expectorate, nature of vomitus, coloring of bruises, depth of lesions, exudate from wounds, nature of rashes. If at all possible, use objective measures. If a photograph is taken it is appropriate to use a tape measure or other object, e.g., a quarter or a pencil, for size comparison.

In written documentation, amounts were often designated as small, moderate, and copious. We now have reasonable, more specific methods to estimate the actual amount of drainage on a dressing or peri-pad, and in many facilities weight scales are used to determine saturation.

---

states that the symptom is of a continuous nature, is the symptom the same all of the time or does it differ in degree? A patient can experience a symptom continuously in duration with differing degrees of strength and severity. Similarly, if the patient declares the symptom to be intermittent in nature, is it regular or irregular in its intermittent occurrence and onset?

In labor and delivery, for example, the nurse clearly measures the laboring woman's contractions for quality, frequency, and duration. The nurse must define the parameters of all symptoms in much the same way even though there may not be a sensitive measurement device such as a fetal monitor to assist in the assessment. Even with the most sophisticated measuring device the patient continues to perceive the symptom based upon past experience, expectation, anxiety levels, and personality.

Whenever you are suggesting possible parameters to a patient, such as "Is the pain there all of the time or some of the time?" you risk introducing biases to the patient. You walk a fine line between investigation and influence. Patients may try to tell you what they believe you want to hear, or what they believe will help the care team successfully treat any given complaint. The nurse is continually estimating and evaluating a patient's response so as to facilitate, but not sway, how a patient will describe what he or she is experiencing.

Mr. X has explained that his pain is dull and burning. Your next inquiry is about any change in the amount of pain related to (r/t) this particular pain episode.

The following sample questions appear in logical order. Remember that a patient's actual answers may distract you from remembering some questions. Re-

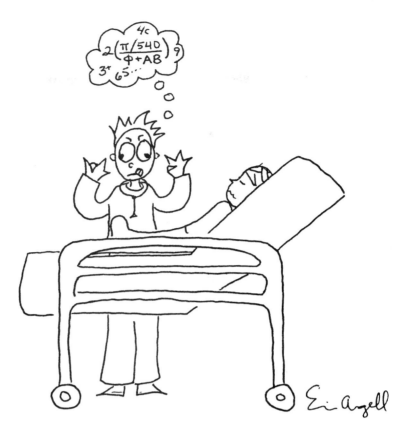

main flexible and listen for answers to your questions in any response the patient might provide.

What made you come to the doctor now?

When did you first notice the change?

On a scale of 1–10, how do you rate your pain?

Is this pain worse than your usual pain?

If so, what makes it worse?

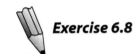

Exercise 6.8

In the following charted notes underline the words that document the quantity characteristic of the given symptom.

Example:

0900: c/o mild, constant, 3/10 pain, onset 0630, anterior border incision site, unrelieved by Tylenol & position Δ.

Answer: constant

1. c/o menstrual cramping and profuse bleeding, 2 pads saturated/hr, × 2 days.

2. Observed scaly erythematous patch, 4 mm × 6 mm, aspect R forearm.

3. Neck—ROM 25° L, 40° R.

4. 3/6 pandiastolic murmur 2nd ICS, L sternal border.

5. c/o intermittent cough, 3–4 episodes per day × 3 days.

> *Case Study 6.1c*
> Charting example: Mr. X
> 1400: c/o "severe, dull, burning" pain; LLQ (abd), 7/10 on 1–10 scale, . . .
> Verbal report
> 1400: c/o severe pain LLQ, 7/10 on 1–10 scale, c̄ Δ from sharp to dull & burning, . . .

CHRONOLOGY

Chronology is related to the timing of a symptom or group of symptoms. When determining the chronology of an event, it may be necessary to begin by asking about broad timing:

"When did you first notice the cough?"

Narrow the time frame to help the patient recall the more specific details: "The cough started two weeks ago as an intermittent problem at night. For the last two days though, the cough has been more continuous and also during the daytime." This is especially helpful if the patient has a long, chronic history with a certain complaint or is experiencing multiple symptoms at the present time of questioning. In cases of emergency you may not be able to solicit any of these details, or you may only be able to obtain a brief, subjective account from a bystander. You will, however, benefit from determining a general time frame and narrowing down the specific details as much as possible.

The timing of a symptom can be instrumental in determining the cause. This is true in exploring environmental or occupational exposure. Stress-related symptoms as well as potential exposures from past travel or group events can

---

BOX 6.7

Chronology

The timing of a symptom and the progression of an observable problem are valuable indicators that can be used in determining a cause and effect relationship. Onset and duration may be linked to events that are often contributors to the underlying problem. You will also be interested in the frequency of occurrence (hourly, daily, monthly), the time of day, the relationship to the work week, and the timing related to meals, fasting, or drinking to determine the progression of a problem.

Often events such as holidays or vacations, or changes perceived as better or worse, will be discovered to trigger an onset of symptoms. A patient may have a pattern of activity that can be related to the onset of a problem. It is interesting to discover patterns in our own behavior that may result in certain outcomes. You may discover a bruise and not remember injuring yourself or notice a topical rash that seems to have come from nowhere. Reviewing your recent activities may help lead you to the onset and subsequent cause of the bruise or rash.

Patients may remember a causative agent when asked to review their usual pattern of activity. A laboratory worker with recurrent eye irritation may benefit by recalling the use of a co-worker's microscope (or sharing other equipment with someone else). The review of the pattern of activity assists in documenting the timing of the event and provides insight into the setting. Be aware of these relationships and look for associations and frequencies.

The words *constant* and *intermittent* are also used to determine chronology. These are good, objective terms that are clearly understood by the patient. A note about a patient who has recently changed jobs to data entry that reads "pain, 8/10, OU, 0400, q noc, M–F × 2 months" demonstrates the effectiveness of documenting the timing of a symptom. People who regularly use computers for long periods are known to have recurrent episodes of eye pain, usually in the middle of the night, but they experience relief on days off. The chronology of the event is instrumental in determining the cause of the problem.

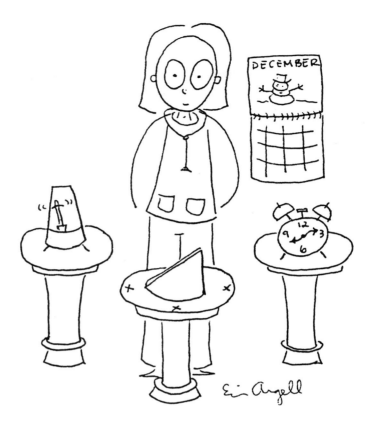

usually be quantified in terms of timing. Epidemiologists can narrow a general outbreak of a disease to the first case and determine how the first patient was exposed as well as the pattern of exposure that occurred afterward with specific and detailed investigations. So too can the nurse isolate the beginning of a symptom with careful inquiry.

With children, and often with adults, relating the onset of a symptom with an event can help narrow the time frame. Holidays, weekends, timing around meals, outings, work, school, or even television shows may be the cues for determining onset, duration, and pattern of a symptom. Is the current illness is a repeat of prior symptoms?

Exercise 6.9

Read the following sentences and circle the words that refer to any chronological relationship:

Example:

Mr. X states that the pain was different after lunch and became increasingly worse until he called you. He said it was like the pain he always experiences when an important business deal is in critical negotiations, and since it always went away in the past he assumed that this would also go away. Instead it intensified until he could not tolerate it.

Answer: after lunch, business deal is in critical negotiations

1. The 2-year-old girl was brought into the office by a child care worker who said that she had been *playing on the floor* happily with the other children when *suddenly she stopped playing* and started to cry while holding the area around her upper right thigh. She *stopped crying for a moment* when her caregiver first

examined the area she was protectively holding. When she was picked up to get into the car to go to the doctors, she *started to cry again and now continues to cry and will not be distracted* from her thigh. She is saying "owwie" and won't let you touch her leg, shrinking back into the child care worker's arms when you approach her.

2. Mrs. Y told the nurse practitioner that through the years, all her periods had been regular and with a 3–4 day cycle of moderate cramps and bleeding. When she began the birth control pills, however, she noticed that her periods seemed to come closer together and with a shorter but much heavier cycle of bleeding and cramping. Sometimes she even has to stay home from work on the first day because the cramps are so uncomfortable.

3. Mr. Z has been on oral hyperglycemic agents for almost ten years and had maintained his blood sugars at a steady level since an attack five years ago which hospitalized him for two days. For a week now he has experienced some flu-like symptoms and tells you he just hasn't been feeling "quite right." He reports a vague feeling of weakness and a sense of nausea "most of the day" and has barely been able to swallow his medications. He notes that he has felt "feverish" for the past two days and this morning when he checked his sugar, it was "extra high."

Case Study 6.1d

Charting example: Mr. X

1400: c/o "severe, dull, burning pain" LLQ (abd), 7/10 on 1–10 scale, onset p̄ lunch, ↑ in severity. Past hx of like pain r/t work. . . .

Verbal report

1400: c/o severe, pain LLQ, 7/10 on 1–10 scale, c̄ Δ from sharp to dull & burning, onset p̄ lunch increasing in intensity. Past history reveals similar episodes at work.

Exercise 6.10

For each of the numbered examples, choose words from the list of descriptors that may be used to modify it.

constant	soft
intermittent	distended
irregular	flat
asymmetrical	round
patchy	equal
dry	rebound
brittle	steady

1. pain _____
2. hair _____
3. eyes _____
4. abdomen _____
5. gait _____
6. wound _____
7. gaze _____

8. skin _____

9. lung sounds _____

10. tenderness _____

SETTING

Like the chronology, the place, context, or setting of the onset of a symptom is important to assess and document. What was the patient doing when they first noticed the symptom? Did the symptom awaken the patient from sleep? Was the patient's symptom associated with a particular activity or ingestion of food? What was the patient's level of stress and exertion when the symptom first developed? The patient may experience a symptom only when in a particular position in or out of bed. The symptom that has its onset toward the middle of the work week and resolves over the weekend is highly suspicious of being a work-related exposure. Symptoms that follow a vacation in a foreign land or other similar experiences may indicate other, additional, exposures.

A classic example of a setting-related symptom based in an overt, external cause is food poisoning. This is especially so if symptoms originate within the context of groups attending the same event. On the other hand, chronically ill persons such as diabetic patients or those with respiratory problems whose symptoms exacerbate need to be asked about the setting in which they noticed problems. The information you elicit related to setting is extremely valuable for treatment of the current problem, prevention of like future episodes, and for possibly determining if a public health problem exists.

BOX 6.8

Setting

As you have seen, the setting in which the onset of the symptom occurs can be key to determining appropriate interventions to implement. In many instances, such as public health, nursing interviews help determine the patient's exposures. Exposure can be related to contacts with like symptoms, as with infectious disease and food poisoning, or environmental exposures, such as smoke, allergens, latex, or chemicals.

Your investigation of the characteristics of a symptom, or observed problem, allows you to use the best nursing skills you have. You will use language to assist a patient to remember the smallest, most minute details that can lead to appropriate health care interventions.

Say a patient reported an increase in pain "after lunch." You need to find out if something happened at lunchtime that caused an increase in pain level, what he ate, if mealtime had preceded other pain episodes. You can help establish a "setting" for the pain episodes that relate to "dull and burning" pain. The setting may end up involving several situations, meals, stress, travel, or you may find that the setting is primarily stress that occurred after lunch. Your attention to these details will help to determine which factors are involved in the pain response and which may be coincidental:

In the past have you had pain after any meals?

Have you had pain when fasting?

Do you remember exactly when you noticed the pain the last time it occurred at work?

Had you eaten?

Is there a particular time of year you have noticed an increase in pain episodes?

Any particular time of day?

How many times has this happened before?

Exercise 6.11

Circle the words that describe the setting of the symptom.

Example:

> Mr. X related to you that the change in symptoms began after lunch, and was like pain he had experienced during important business situations.
>
> ***Answer: lunch, business situations***

1. Mrs. X stated that her son always had stomach complaints mid-week after PE.
2. Ms. T stated that she runs 5 mi qod but only has breathing problems in midwinter.
3. Mr. H stated that he and his family have a good relationship and that his feelings of anxiety only seem to occur during the winter months.
4. Seven employees were admitted from the office one week after the office was painted and fumigated.
5. Mr. M's back pain gets worse when he is walking laps at the mall.

Case Study 6.1e

Charting example: Mr. X

1400: c/o "severe, dull, burning pain"; LLQ (abd), 7/10 on 1–10 scale, onset $\bar{p}$ lunch, ↑ in severity. Past hx of pain r/t work, 5–6/year × 2 yr., always $\bar{p}$ business meals . . .

Verbal report

1400: c/o severe, pain LLQ, 7/10 on 1–10 scale, $\bar{c}$ Δ from sharp to dull & burning, onset $\bar{p}$ lunch increasing in intensity. Past history reveals similar episodes with work-related meal meetings . . .

ASSOCIATED MANIFESTATIONS

While interviewing the patient about the primary or chief complaint, you may also need to explore what if any other symptoms are concurrent with the patient's presenting complaint. Questions related to associated manifestations are frequently formulated during the interview about additional sensations or feelings related to the primary reason for the patient's visit. For instance a patient with severe headaches may note visual disturbance and nausea as well. These related symptoms, while not the primary source of discomfort for the patient, may provide clues in determining the root cause of the problem. An interviewer may also ask about pertinent positive or negative findings in an effort to establish the basis for the patient's complaint. For example, a patient may be asked about the presence of bloody or tarry stools associated with complaints of changing bowel habits. A concurrent complaint may also be unrelated to the primary problem; avoid discounting complaints that appear unrelated.

At times, associated manifestations may be related to the patient's attitude or mood and are not necessarily based in physical findings. Depression and fear are important to note, as is euphoria. Cardiac patients have been noted to experience "feelings of impending doom" related to the onset of a cardiac episode.

Associated manifestations may overlap with the elements of timing and setting. A patient whose complaint is related to pain with meals may also have ac-

BOX 6.9

Associated Manifestations

Dealing with the category of associated manifestations or symptoms is often very confusing for the beginner. It is frankly an issue for experienced nurses. You must remember that you are not determining a medical diagnosis (unless you are a nurse practitioner). Instead you are compiling a list of symptoms experienced by a patient that may or may not be related to the presenting problem or chief complaint.

For example, migraine headaches are often associated with visual disturbance, vertigo, and nausea. These associated manifestations may support the diagnosis of "migraine" but their absence does not rule out (r/o) migraines. An experienced interviewer will also ask a patient about "visual" changes, events, or disturbances rather than the typical "aura." The patient will then be free to offer their interpretations of any possible visual event, such as diplopia (double vision), floaters, photophobia, or aura. You are less likely to bias the patient by asking a broader question when relevant than by singling out specific possibilities.

Other areas of questioning will often refer to "constitutional" symptoms such as energy, appetite, and well-being. If you introduce the word *fatigue* with a positive response from your patient it may lead to the provider ordering of a battery of tests that are unlikely to benefit the patient. Fatigue is a diagnosis as well as a symptom; the word itself implies that the patient may need further assessment. If the patient introduces the word, it should be in quotes with a complete description of what "fatigue" means to the patient, how it manifests, and what effect it is having on daily activities. Don't ignore this complaint, but do avoid putting words in the patient's mouth.

companying bloating or gastric discomfort. The presence of hyperactive bowel sounds, occurring in the time frame of a symptom event is an example of this seeming overlap. Carefully dissected, the bowel sound is the *associated symptom*, meals represent the *setting*, and the *chronology* is noted in determining if the hyperactive bowel sound precedes or follows eating.

Exercise 6.12

Consider the following samples and select those words or phrases that indicate a potential as associated symptoms in the patient's history of the complaint.

Example:

Mr. X adds that on prior occasions he had noticed "bloating" and loud embarrassing "stomach growling" along with the pain sensation but had no feelings of nausea. He did state that he had a hard time getting "regular" bowel movements, often alternating between constipation and diarrhea.

Answer: hyperactive bowel sounds, irregular bowel movements, bloating

1. Ms. Y presented to the doctor's office wearing sunglasses indoors. She states that she cannot tolerate light now because she is having "the worst headache of her life." She also complains of decreased food intake because of nausea but has had no vomiting. The headache is a constant, stabbing pain, which seems to be stronger over her right eye. She has tried numerous over-the-counter medications but has experienced no relief. Ms. Y tells you that the headache started two days ago, "has never been relieved," and is "getting worse by the minute." She also states she doesn't know "how much longer she can stand it" and that now, when she stands up, she "feels dizzy from the pain."

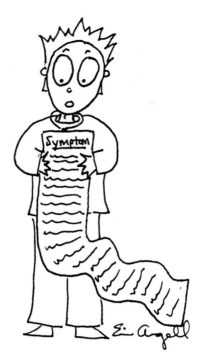

"Mom always said you are judged by who you associate with."

2. Mr. Z presents to the emergency department with his family stating that he thinks he had a "seizure" because he experienced an episode of "blacking out." He was working in the fields as a laborer when he felt an overwhelming need to sit down before he "fainted." His family reports to you that once before Mr. Z seemed to "drift off," stopped a conversation he was involved in at the time, and then began a gentle but overall rhythmic shaking in both of his arms. The shaking in his arms lasted about 10 seconds and then progressed to include a more violent shaking of Mr. Z's "entire body" which lasted a full minute. When the activity stopped, Mr. Z's family noticed that he had "peed his pants" and also seemed to be "dazed" for a while after with no clear memory of the event's sequence. Shortly after he went into his room and laid down and slept heavily for two hours.

Exercise 6.13

Choose which are most likely associated symptoms in the following histories and word them for clarity.

1. Your patient, admitted for a fractured L hip, tells you she has had several fainting episodes and needs to eat frequent small meals due to headaches. She misses her evening cocktail and is anxious about canceling her weekly cleaning service.

2. Lucy J., 16 y/o, admitted for malnutrition, states she stopped menstruating 3 months ago. She is inactive and does not participate in after school activities. Her grades are average, although she tested as a gifted student. She states she used marijuana twice at parties.

3. Mr. P, a farm worker, presents at the ER c/o N, V, & D × 4 days. You observe him scratching his arms. His skin is dry and has poor turgor. He asks for water and a wet cloth to clean the dirt from his face.

4. Ms. B is admitted with a diagnosis of severe depression. She does not fill out her meal choices and spends her time pacing and looking out the window. She asks for all calls to be diverted.

5. James is being worked up for rapid weight gain r/t thyroid disease. He c/o the frigid temperature in the office. His blood pressure is 90/58, pulse 62, and states he is too tired to do any exercise.

Case Study 6.1f

Charting example: Mr. X

1400: c/o "severe, dull, burning pain"; LLQ (abd), 7/10 on 1–10 scale, onset p̄ lunch, ↑ in severity. Past hx of pain r/t work, 5–6/year × 2 yr., always p̄ business meals, c̄ bloating & hyperresonant bowel sounds, alternating diarrhea & constipation, . . .

Verbal report

1400: c/o severe, pain LLQ, 7/10 on 1–10 scale, c̄ (from sharp to dull & burning, onset p̄ lunch increasing in intensity. Past history reveals similar episodes associated with work-related meal meetings. Symptoms include bloating & hyperresonant bowel sounds, alternating diarrhea & constipation, . . .

ALLEVIATING/AGGRAVATING FACTORS

The characteristic of alleviating and/or aggravating factors is specifically about actions by the patient that make the presenting symptom feel better or feel worse. Interventions include prescription medicines, over-the-counter (OTC) remedies, quantity and type of meals, and assuming certain positions. A patient may also change personal health habits, environmental factors, spirituality, alternative treatments, conventional treatment, or activity levels to improve their symptoms.

During the interview you have an opportunity to evaluate the patient's responses as to the nature, degree, severity and impact the patient's complaint carries.

BOX 6.10

Alleviating/Aggravating Factors

Alleviating factors change the patient's presenting complaint by lessening the symptoms. They make the patient feel better. Position of comfort, activity, diet, fasting, prescription (Rx) drugs, over-the-counter (OTC) medications, vitamins, alternative remedies and treatments, biofeedback, physical therapy, prayer, and meditation are all worthy of being documented.

Aggravating factors are those that increase the problem or make it worse. All of the previously mentioned categories are included. Even the most appropriate interventions can "do harm" if the patient responds poorly to it.

A good example that demonstrates the character of alleviating or aggravating factors is activity level. Activity and exercise are recommended for a healthy cardiovascular system. However, exercise exacerbates congestive heart failure (CHF). Patients with diabetes and asthma must monitor and regulate activity levels. A patient who is obese must incorporate exercise into the daily regimen. Besides being factors that affect the status of a patient's symptom, activity and exercise also are interactive and necessary to the baseline health of most patients.

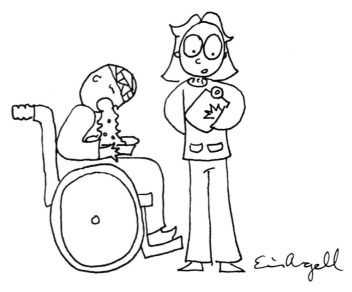

"Hmmm . . . sitting up makes your nausea worse."

Your questions will guide the patient's response to the symptom in question but the patient may easily interpret your introductory questions to have a broader meaning. It is up to you to listen carefully and to learn to differentiate effectively. Record a factual accounting of the patient's subjective description of any contributing information about the symptom (or about the effectiveness of treatment).

Have you heard the statement "the devil is in the details"? When interviewing a patient about their complaints or about the effectiveness of interventions it is best to heed these words. The amount and level of detail you can elicit from a patient, relevant to the primary complaint can make a difference. Patients with a poor response to medical intervention may be better able to understand and accept the limitations of their care if they feel that the health care team has sought appropriate information as to what the patient perceives contributes to their problem. The best medical results can be tainted by the patient's feeling that they have been only a body or number in an assembly line treatment plant.

Exercise 6.14

Identify the categories of aggravating and or alleviating factors in the following scenarios:

Example:

Mr. X continues by stating that he never used any medications not prescribed by the doctor. He said his secretary would bring him hot tea and within a few hours he would feel "much better." You find out through careful questioning that the tea is an herbal "concoction" and that Mr. X always keeps antacid tablets in his desk. Mr. X also says that he is more comfortable when he reclines with his knees bent.

Answer: Alleviated by OTC medications, alternative treatment, position

1. Mrs. C presents with c/o back pain. She recalls no specific incident or injury. She sits at work doing phone sales and data entry. At home she likes to participate in computer chat room discussions and does gardening. She says she has tried all OTC medications with no relief. She recalls she used to take walks at

lunchtime but she changed jobs during the rainy season and prefers to eat at her desk and read.

2. Mr. D reports that he thinks he has gallbladder problems. He c/o midgastric pain that radiates to his R shoulder. He has been avoiding fatty foods and is eating salads regularly but is not feeling better. He also wakes in the night with heartburn and takes baking soda for relief. He says it helps a little. He drinks coffee throughout the day with no problems falling asleep.

3. Mr. H, who is in CHF (congestive heart failure), presents with shortness of breath. He takes diuretics and digoxin. He says that he has limited his fluids to 2 cups of coffee/day and sips of water, because he gets dizzy each time he gets up to urinate. He also feels as if he wants to throw up. He is on oxygen, which helps him rest comfortably.

MEANING TO PATIENT

The meaning of the problem, to the patient, is a much more personal aspect of the complaint. Finding out how patients feel about their illness, symptoms, and the impact of the ongoing treatment experience on their well-being is vital information. Illness can deprive a patient of income, social standing, hobbies, and leisure activities. It can also greatly affect self-respect and personal sense of well-being.

In the ROS assessment interview, you may hear caregivers judge a patient's responses by saying the patient does not want to be well. There are some people whose "well-being" may rely on the attention derived from illness, who benefit from being sick. However, this is not a frequent response by patients. When questioning the patient about the meaning or impact of their problem, be neutral to any response they might offer. It may be a sensitive area for patients to discuss and often indicates a sense of trust in their caregiver to reveal such personal information.

The patient who remains undiagnosed, that is, one who experiences illness but does not know the specific cause, will often be relieved even by a grave

---

BOX 6.11

Meaning to Patient

This category is another that overlaps with many of the earlier categories, but can also explore effects on a patient's life that may not be as obvious to the interviewer. For example, in some states those on state assistance can only collect their monthly check in person. The economic effect of illness can devastate a family. Skilled nursing residents can lose their "home" after using up life's savings paying for care needs and be moved to a facility that is less desirable or to which the family has restricted access due to location.

Economics, social status, past experiences, family obligations, and work environment all contribute to a patient's personal response to any threat to their usual status and well-being. Medical problems need not be life-threatening to affect a patient's life or livelihood. Pregnancy is a perfect example of a "normal" condition that requires nursing intervention; it may have been planned or unplanned, the woman may know the father of the baby or not. Although a "normal" condition, pregnancy's meaning to the individual woman and family can vary tremendously.

As you question the patient, you may find the patient returning vague answers to a direct question such as "How is this affecting your life?" or "How do you feel about that?" There may be more subtle references to the effect on the patient's well-

(continued on next page)

BOX 6.11—*Continued*

being throughout the interview, and you will need to listen for key words and phrases. As you listen, you can try to open a dialogue about life changes with the individual patient, but realize that many patients prefer not to speculate about these issues with anyone, let alone with a relative stranger.

A good example is the patient who mentions that a neighbor is feeding his or her pets during this hospitalization. This comment can disclose concerns about the overall well-being of the animals or even that they are concerned about lack of family support. If the patient is relying on a neighbor and has no immediate family nearby, the implications are different than for a patient who has family members who are not helping out. The specific data regarding these situations alter the concerns. These may be further altered by the patient's perception of the circumstances. You will also be filtering the information to determine what, if any, interventions are necessary and available in each individual case.

Take care and show respect when gathering this very personal information. If you are severely time-limited and cannot refer to social services or pastoral care for follow-up, you are at risk for exposing a patient's deepest fears and creating increased vulnerability. The psychosocial issues are important enough to be included in the review of systems and need to be addressed in a serious manner. They are not merely a symptom characteristic. They are an integral component of wellness of "body, mind, and spirit."

Key words and phrases to be aware of include: afraid, it doesn't matter, home concerns ranging from family obligations to houseplants, afford, job loss, insurance coverage, mistrust of health care team, don't tell my family.

Body language indicating withdrawal during the interview such as changes in eye contact, assertive or aggressive responses, turning away, and striking out are indicators that the patient may not be able to address their concerns with you at this time. Respect the space the patient may be asking for but share your observations with the patient's medical provider so as not to disregard important signals.

diagnosis. It is difficult for human beings to face the unknown, and fear can become an overwhelming element in the process. If from your specific and detailed assessment a diagnosis is able to be determined, it may likely provide overwhelming relief for your patient. In determining the efficacy of a treatment, your

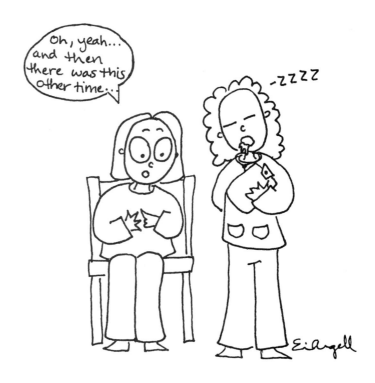

data could potentially lead to determining a more successful treatment modality. The importance of good investigation cannot be overemphasized.

Case Study 6.1g

In reviewing Mr. X's history you note that his past history (PH) of symptoms (sx) occur with greater frequency during business meetings, which often include lunch. He trusted his secretary when she offered him tea that seemed to relieve his symptoms. It appears as though he is very concerned about the impact any illness would have on his work schedule.

PUTTING THE PIECES TOGETHER

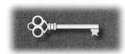

Communication involves spoken words, body language, and a contractual agreement to share information. Documentation relies wholly on the written word. The language of your documentation must clearly describe the situation. Verbal reports may be affected by the relationship between caregivers, so written words must succinctly state the information necessary to eliminate, as much as possible, the potential for interpretive error.

Soliciting information from the patient will likely depend on a nurse's knowing the correct way to ask a question, by restating the question using words more understandable by the patient, and by having the patient restate the problem using his or her own words. A direct patient quote *may* be necessary if there is no better way to describe the response without changing its meaning. Include objective information where possible to support the documentation and help validate your documentation.

It helps to break the assessment questions down into a number of clear specific points, rather than asking broad, general questions. If a patient can answer yes or no to some of the questions, he or she may be more likely to offer more complete details as necessary. Remember, take care to avoid leading the patient to answer a question a certain way or to offer words the patient might use. Let the patient use his or her own words to respond.

Case Study 6.2

Read the following scenario. List the pertinent information included under each of the descriptor categories. Choose appropriate descriptors and practice charting as you would in a nursing narrative. If there seems to be no appropriate or apparent descriptor, then consider using a direct quote from the patient.

Hint: use your dictionary or nursing text if data is presented that you do not understand.

Lucy B. is a 68-year-old woman who was admitted for bilateral pneumonia. She has been undergoing chemotherapy for lymphoma for one year and has had several episodes of respiratory-related illness, most notably five visits to her MD in the past month with complaint of bronchitis. VS are 102°F (o), BP: 120/80; AP: 95; RR: 24; O2 sat: 88% on room air. She is sitting with her upper body bent forward and appears to be "reaching" for air. Her skin is pale and damp with a slight bluish tinge around the lips and nares. She is holding her hands together tightly below her sternum. She states that her "stomach is upset." When she speaks you observe that her mouth and oral membranes are dry and caked with cloudy, green-tinged, dry sputum, which she occasionally tries to wipe away with a tissue.

Her husband of 45 years remarks that she has been coughing for 3 weeks but has resisted visiting her provider. She has also been refusing help with the daily chores that she has been doing for the duration of their marriage. He does acknowledge that he has been helping with food preparation such as potato peeling and chopping vegetables, but she has been refusing to allow her adult children to assist in any cleaning task or gardening.

One of her daughters takes you aside to tell you that her mother has been discussing her desired funeral arrangements. She states that her mother feels like she has become useless and a burden to the family. The daughter confides that the family has been trying to help Lucy feel comfortable and that they have brought an extra bed into the living area and arranged pillows for her so that she can feel comfortable and stay involved with daily activities. She only agrees to this arrangement when she is too exhausted to do "her housework."

General Appearance

Location

Quality

Quantity

Chronology

Setting

Associated Manifestations

Aggravating/Alleviating Factors

Meaning to Patient

Written Narrative Charting for Case Study 6.2

Answer Guide

Exercise 6.1

1. local
   Common: person from a particular area; branch of labor union
   Technical: not general or systemic anesthetic limited to one area

2. exquisite
   Common: elaborately done; beautiful
   Technical: intense, keen, sharp

3. persistent
   Common: enduring; continuing firmly in spite of obstacle
   Technical: obstinate continuation, despite the environmental conditions

4. advanced
   Common: highly developed; complex
   Technical: far along in course

5. vegetative
   Common: relating to plants or plant growth; capable of growth
   Technical: not active; growing or functioning involuntarily or unconsciously

6. reversible
   Common: turned backward in position, order, or direction
   Technical: turning in opposite direction of disease, symptom, or state

7. loose
   Common: not tightly fastened, bound, stapled, or bundled; not exact in interpretation; demonstrating lack of restraint; immoral
   Technical: not formed or bound together in reference to stool or tissue; mental associations implying disordered thought process

8. murmur
   Common: low continuous sound; mutter
   Technical: soft sound heard while listening to heart or vessels

9. injection
   Common: forcing one element (gas or liquid) into another (ground); introducing a subject into a discussion
   Technical: introducing medicine into tissue or vein; congestion or hyperemia, as with a red eye

10. boring
    Common: dull; repetitive
    Technical: drilling or digging sensation

11. pounding
    Common: striking repeatedly; crushing by forceful beating
    Technical: heavy throbbing sensation

12. thready
    Common: having to do with fibrous strands twisted together; ridges on screws or bolts; common element that is cohesive
    Technical: description of pulse quality that is weaker and fairly rapid, often indicating hypovolemia

13. excursion
    Common: short trip or outing usually for pleasure; digression
    Technical: deviation from expected normal course

14. quadrant
    Common: altitude determining instrument; mathematical plane
    Technical: division of an anatomical region for purpose of description

15. mass
    Common: nonspecific quantity or amount of matter; reference to greatest number of members of common group; religious celebration
    Technical: number of cells grouped together, such as tumor; physical properties of matter that give it measurable dimensions

16. rebound
    Common: bounce or spring back; recover after a let down
    Technical: sudden contraction of muscle after relaxation; sudden response to an activity or treatment after the stimulus has been removed

17. dilate
    Common: enlarge or expand
    Technical: enlarge cavity either through intention, disease process, or normal response

18. anterior
    Common: front location
    Technical: reference in anatomical position to areas facing forward

19. ribbon
    Common: narrow strip of cloth or decorative fabric
    Technical: stool formed flat and narrow

Exercise 6.2

1. unilateral
   assigning condition or symptom to singular side of body or specific part of body

2. bilateral
   condition or symptom that is observed to occur equally or unequally on both sides of the body or a part of the body

3. anterior
   in anatomical position referring to any part of the body that faces front

4. posterior
   in anatomical position referring to any part of the body that faces back

5. aspect
   appearance or position that faces a designated direction

6. upper
   location of designated part that is highest in position

7. outer
   that which is away from the center of the body part or body in anatomical reference

8. quadrants
   division of a circle (or specified part of anatomy) into 4 equal sections of 90° where they meet

9. inner
   that which is located near to the center of the body or body part referenced

10. midline
    line which divides the body or a part of the body in half

11. symmetry
    balance demonstrated by comparing two sides of a single structure or both components of a pair of same structures or parts

12. supine
    body positioned flat on back

13. prone
    body positioned flat on abdomen with head positioned straight or facing in either direction

14. measurement
    objective determination of dimensions or features

15. mid-
    prefix referencing the center of object

16. left
    side that faces north when front of object faces east

17. right
    opposite of left or side that faces south when front of object faces east

18. proximal
    reference nearest to the point of origin, such as trunk or hand

19. distal
    farthest away from point of origin

20. sub-
    prefix for beneath or under

Exercise 6.3

1. periorbital
2. submandibular
3. midclavicular
4. axillary
5. midsternal
6. midepigastric
7. umbilical
8. suprapubic
9. distal femoral
10. anterior patellar

Exercise 6.4

1. b;   2. c;   3. b;   4. a;   5. c

Exercise 6.5

1. bilaterally
2. intact
3. absent
4. equal
5. round
6. reactive
7. light
8. warm
9. dry
10. accommodation

Exercise 6.6

1. Pupils are equal, round, and reactive to light and accommodation.
2. Dressing is intact.
3. Skin is warm and dry.
4. Pedal pulse is palpable bilaterally.
5. Reflex is absent left lower extremity (LLE).

Exercise 6.7

1. stabbing, sensitive
2. ringing
3. serosanguineous, multiple
4. granulation, redness, swelling
5. rapid, apex
6. labored, dusky
7. full, pressure

8. numbness, tingling
9. pale, cool
10. sharp, exquisite

Exercise 6.8

1. 2 pads saturated/hr
2. 4 mm $\times$ 6 mm
3. 25° L, 40° R
4. pandiastolic
5. 3–4 episodes per day

Exercise 6.9

1. playing on the floor, suddenly she stopped playing, stopped crying for a moment, started to cry again and now continues to cry and will not be distracted
2. all her periods had been regular, when began the birth control pills, come closer together, shorter but much heavier cycle, so uncomfortable.
3. ten years, blood sugars at a steady level, for a week, flu-like symptoms, feeling of weakness, sense of nausea, felt "feverish" for the past two days, this morning, was "extra high"

Exercise 6.10

1. pain: constant; intermittent; rebound; irregular; steady
2. hair: patchy; dry; brittle
3. eyes: asymmetrical; flat; round; equal
4. abdomen: irregular; soft; distended; flat; round; equal; rebound
5. gait: asymmetrical; steady
6. wound: irregular; patchy; dry
7. gaze: constant; irregular; steady
8. skin: patchy; dry; brittle; soft
9. lung sounds: intermittent; constant; equal
10. tenderness: constant; intermittent; rebound

Exercise 6.11

1. after PE
2. runs 5 mi, midwinter
3. winter months
4. office
5. walking laps at the mall

Exercise 6.12

1. cannot tolerate light, decreased food intake because of nausea, feels dizzy from the pain
2. need to sit down before he "fainted," "drift off," shaking in both of his arms, "peed his pants," "dazed," no clear memory, slept heavily

Exercise 6.13

1. eating pattern, fainting, alcohol, headaches
2. inactivity, change in academic achievement, menstrual cessation
3. dry skin, pruritis, thirst, poor turgor
4. without appetite, restlessness, isolation
5. cold intolerance, hypotension, bradycardia, lethargy

Exercise 6.14

1. alleviated by walking, aggravated by sitting
2. aggravated by diet and caffeine intake, alleviated slightly by bicarbonate
3. aggravated by ↓ fluid volume, alleviated by oxygen, rest

CHAPTER 7

Systems, Descriptors, and Documentation

WORD LIST

block	output	expire
relief	stream	reduce
trigger	tremors	
intake	fixation	

 Exercise 7.1

Each item in the word list has both common and technical meanings. Match each word with its corresponding set of definitions and compare the intent or usage of the terms as both common and technical words.

1. _____
   Common: trembling as in slight earth shaking
   Technical: body movement that is involuntary, usually a slight tremble can be regular or intermittent

2. _____
   Common: amount of work, energy, or product produced within a time frame
   Technical: quantity of urine, excretion, or other measured substance over a given period

3. _____
   Common: strong attachment or obsession
   Technical: being immobilized and firmly attached; preserving tissue sample for analysis

4. _____
   Common: body of water running in channel of earth's surface
   Technical: steady flow of liquid, especially urine

5. _____
   Common: a taking in; place in a pipe where water is taken in
   Technical: amount of food or fluid absorbed by patient

6. _____
   Common: solid section of wood usually with flat sides; section of a city with defined parameters
   Technical: interruption in the transmission of impulse, e.g., cardiac or nerve

7. _____
   Common: come to an end; to die
   Technical: breathe out; to die

8. _____

   Common: lessening of discomfort; aid given to needy; art or map with elevated components

   Technical: alleviation of symptom; area under prosthesis intended to reduce pressure

9. _____

   Common: lessen or diminish

   Technical: restore by manipulation or surgery to normal position

10. _____

    Common: a release for discharging a firearm

    Technical: a stimulus for a physiological or chemical event

SYSTEMS APPROACH

You are now ready to focus on documenting from the time of a patient's being admitted to the hospital to the moment of discharge. This will be accomplished with the use of progressive case studies. You will begin with the admitting assessment and document your assessment of the patient's progress. The case studies are based on usual and ordinary hospital and clinic experiences. Each of the key concepts from previous chapters will be represented, and all body systems will be included to provide practical charting experience.

Begin the first case study. The answer guide at the end of the chapter provides charting examples for you to compare with your own. We recommend that you check these pages after you have completed your own charting.

It is not necessary for your charting to be exactly the same as the text. If there are differences, however, you should be prepared to justify your choices (are your priorities in the best interest of the patient?) and validate to yourself that your documentation stands the test of time (will you understand what you meant in 5 years?).

Note: The case studies are purposefully incomplete. While working with the case studies, you are likely to feel that you need more information than what is offered. Remember the case studies are not teaching nursing process and you need to chart known information. However, the link between proper charting and good nursing care will become apparent as you recognize the deficiency of data. In actual clinical experience much data are collected over an extended time period and added to the general database.

Good luck with the case studies!

Case Study 7.1a

You are admitting Mrs. F, a 75-year-old widow with a 10-year history of diverticulitis, who lives alone in a retirement community. Her friend convinced her to see a physician after Mrs. F confided that she had been having "severe stomach pain" that caused her to "double up," was "constipated," was unable to have more than a trickle for a bowel movement, and had eaten only broth for three days. She had also been quite embarrassed by loud gurgling sounds "from her stomach." She is treating herself with Bactrim, which she obtained from friends who regularly visit Mexico. She was prescribed this medication whenever she had a "flare up" of diverticulitis in the past. She continued to self-medicate when her insurance changed and she had to choose a new primary care provider.

She was seen in the acute clinic by an unfamiliar physician who did a cursory history. He took the precaution of doing an abdominal X-ray, which indicated that there was a probability of bowel obstruction. Endoscopy confirmed the presence of obstruction; although Mrs. F. felt that she was "not sick." She was referred to a surgeon and subsequently agreed to be admitted to the hospital for further examination, antibiotic therapy, and nutritional support.

She is admitted on your shift with no supporting history and physical, and no previous admits for reference. You are to complete the admitting history and physical assessment.

1. Prioritize the objective and subjective data for written documentation.

   OBJECTIVE   SUBJECTIVE

   _____   _____

   _____   _____

   _____   _____

   _____   _____

   _____   _____

   _____   _____

   _____   _____

2. Using the CHH format, record known data as you would in a patient record.

   _____

   _____

   _____

   _____

3. List the data that are relevant and should be prioritized in history gathering.

   _____

   _____

   _____

   _____

4. Which key concepts are represented in your answer?

   _____

   _____

   _____

   _____

Case Study 7.1b

During the admitting interview you learn that Mrs. F has been in general good health all of her life and has had few reasons to visit a physician. In fact, she has had no screening tests done which are indicated for a female in her age group nor has she been active regarding health promotion or disease prevention.

Because she has been admitted for possible surgery you determine that you need to prioritize the issues necessary for her to be treated safely during this hospital visit.

Among the details you feel compelled to address are a 55-year smoking history and the daily use of alcohol. A nutrition history is also indicated to assess her general health status related to the history and duration of the bowel obstruction.

You will also be monitoring IV antibiotic therapy, MS 10 mg prn, hyperalimentation via PIKK line, and output via Foley catheter. With the exception of ice chips Mrs. F is NPO.

Mrs. F still insists she does not feel sick, has no pain, and should not even be in the hospital. You know that her admitting diagnosis indicates that she is likely to have a bowel resection and a colostomy. It is not known if the colostomy is more likely to be temporary or permanent. You feel that a mental health assessment is appropriate and decide on the nursing diagnoses that are appropriate for this patient. Your documentation needs to support your decision.

1.   What data would you consider in choosing the nursing diagnosis "Knowledge deficit related to health maintenance and disease prevention"?

_____

_____

_____

_____

2.   What key concepts might be useful in assessing health maintenance problems?

_____

_____

_____

3.   What data would you consider in choosing the nursing diagnosis "Knowledge deficit r/t effective management of diverticulitis"?

_____

_____

_____

_____

Case Study 7.1c

Mrs. F is on her first day postop hemicolectomy with colostomy. She refers to the colostomy as "this thing" but watches you as you check the bag and inspect her dressing. She says she accepts that the procedure was necessary and is comforted by the fact that the surgeon assured her that the colostomy will be temporary. She makes good eye contact throughout your visit.

She states she wants to go home because she is tired of being in the hospital. She does not resist ambulation, although she moves slowly with a hesitant gait. You ask if she is in pain and she states "only when getting out of bed or when I cough." You remember that she also stated that she was not in pain preoperatively and are concerned that she may be denying pain. You check vital signs to determine if she has increased HR or BP and find that her vital signs have been stable.

You are to arrange for her to have home visits from the enterostomal nursing staff and believe that you need to clearly convey that Mrs. F has been receptive to learning how to perform self-care and that her goal is to be prepared for the take down surgery as soon as it is medically possible. You write the discharge note after you make sure that there will be someone to help care for her in her home.

1.   With the available data, write an objective discharge assessment that describes Mrs. F's adjustment to the colostomy.

_____

_____

_____

_____

Case Study 7.2a

You admit a 55-year-old male, Mr. D, who presented at the emergency department with difficulty breathing. He states no history of smoking or cardiopulmonary disorders. Vital signs are BP 140/80, HR 120, R 30, T 98.6°F, O_2 sat 90%. He is restless, and slightly diaphoretic but states no chest pain or discomfort other than breathing difficulty. He says he had "hay fever" as a child that was noticeable from April through October and was managed by OTC antihistamines. He has not needed medication for almost 30 years. Lung X-ray reveals normal lung tissue with no infiltrates. There are bronchial wheezes noted through auscultation, greater with forced expiration. Preliminary diagnosis is reactive airway disease (RAD).

You have no information regarding any other potential exposures, because the immediate respiratory interventions took priority. He was medicated with a bronchodilator in the ER and is on 2 l/m O_2 by cannula. You observe that he is more comfortable positioned at 45°, is not pale or dusky and that his O_2 is now at 95%.

You decide to complete some of his health history to see if you can determine the possible cause of the respiratory dysfunction. You begin by asking him when he first noticed that his breathing was changed. He states that he was taking his usual walk at lunchtime when he noticed he was short of breath. He returned to his office and could not "catch his breath." A co-worker noticed his distress and notified employee health, and the paramedics were called.

You are aware that the temperatures outside are unseasonably cold and that the wind is a factor in making the air even chillier and drier. Knowing that there is a relationship between RAD and exercising in these weather conditions you consider that the conditions may be a contributing environmental cause to his problem.

1. Prioritize the objective and subjective data for written documentation.

   OBJECTIVE   SUBJECTIVE

   _____   _____
   _____   _____
   _____   _____
   _____   _____
   _____   _____
   _____   _____
   _____   _____
   _____   _____
   _____   _____

2. Write a verbal report for presentation to the nursing instructor.

   _____
   _____
   _____
   _____

3. Write an admitting note using CHH format.

   _____
   _____
   _____
   _____

Case Study 7.2b

Mr. D. had no critical events during the night. He appeared to be resting comfortably in semi-Fowlers position through the night. He aroused easily for routine checks of vital signs. His pulse ox improved to 98% and his skin was warm and dry with capillary refill of two seconds. His color was good, no pursed lip breathing was observed. He was able to ambulate to the bathroom and stated that the symptoms had not returned. His lung sounds were clear with no wheeze on forced expiration. VS: R decreased to 20 & apical HR to 80.

1. State the objective findings that you include in the end of shift documentation.

   _____

   _____

   _____

   _____

2. Write a verbal report for presentation to the nursing instructor.

   _____

   _____

   _____

   _____

Case Study 7.2c

The provider discharges the patient to home with instructions to return to the office for a thorough examination on the following Monday. He tells Mr. D that he may return to work but to wait until after his follow-up checkup to resume his exercise routine. You are given the responsibility to complete discharge teaching.

   In your instructions you include: follow physician's instructions, return to the clinic for follow-up, and seek help if the symptoms return prior to the visit. You suggest that he might try to recall any similar events and reconstruct the circumstances in which they occurred as well as what relieved similar symptoms in the past. You ask him if he can repeat back the instructions to you. Satisfied that he appears to understand his follow-up plan you complete the discharge.

1. Write a discharge note.

   _____

   _____

   _____

   _____

Case Study 7.3a

The emergency room nurse has transported a new patient to ICU Room 2 by gurney. The patient is Ms. T, a 17-year-old female with an admitting diagnosis of acetaminophen overdose. As you assist the ER nurse in moving Ms. T from gurney to bed, the RN gives you the following information: the patient has a history of two previous overdoses; she lives with her mother, who is single; her vital signs are pulse 80, respirations 12, BP 100/50; she arrived via ambulance to the ER and has been lethargic but arousable and is otherwise oriented × 3; her mother came home from work this evening and found her on the living room couch, unarousable, with an empty bottle of Tylenol on the floor next to her. The ER RN tells you that Ms. T also has a boyfriend who, according to the mother, treats Ms. T. "really well." The RN also tells you that she received 1 g activated charcoal lavage per NG, which was subsequently removed.

1. Prioritize the objective and subjective data for written documentation.

   OBJECTIVE   SUBJECTIVE

   _____   _____
   _____   _____
   _____   _____
   _____   _____
   _____   _____
   _____   _____
   _____   _____

2. Write a verbal report for presentation to the nursing instructor.

   _____
   _____
   _____
   _____

3. Write an admitting note using CHH format.

   _____
   _____
   _____
   _____

Case Study 7.3b

At 1800 you assess Ms. T and obtain more data. Although quite lethargic, she awakens when you say her name and is able to answer your questions in complete sentences. Her neurological assessment yields the following data: PERRLA, MAE, no unilateral weakness. Speech is clear and coherent.
VS: T 37.4°F, P 60, R 14, BP 90/50.
Other observations:
An IV of D5.45%NS is infusing at 100 cc/h. No open wounds. No visible scars. Denies nausea. Tongue is midline, w/ black discoloration. Pt. states she had her period "about 3 weeks ago." She denies the use of recreational or prescription drugs. She says that she has been "depressed" lately because her boyfriend has a new job and has been "ignoring" her. Dr. L is her family physician; she states, "he's nice, but he doesn't know anything. . . ."

1. Write a follow-up narrative for the chart.

   _____
   _____
   _____
   _____

Case Study 7.4a

You are working evening shift in the cardiac transitional unit. Your patient, Mr. C, had a cardiac catheterization today. He returned from the cath lab at 1400. You assess him at 1545. Upon entering the room, you find a drowsy, pleasant, 58-year-old man in no visible distress. You ask if he has any discomfort, and he responds that "he feels fine." His EKG monitor shows sinus rhythm. He has a 7 French arterial sheath in his right groin. The sheath site is soft and without drainage. His pedal pulses are 2+ bilaterally. VS: HR 80, R 14, BP 136/70. He has an IV of NS at 100 cc/hr. His lung sounds are clear bilaterally.

He asks if he can lie on his side. You explain that he needs to keep his right leg straight because of the sheath in his groin.

1. Prioritize the objective and subjective data for written documentation.

OBJECTIVE   SUBJECTIVE

_____   _____

_____   _____

_____   _____

_____   _____

_____   _____

_____   _____

2. Write a verbal report for presentation to the nursing instructor.

3. Write an admitting note.

Case Study 7.4b

You have recorded your initial assessment. Upon returning to Mr. C's room at 1700, you find that he has turned onto his right side. "My back was really hurting. Being on my side helps," he states. "I kind of feel like I am urinating, though."

1. What subjective symptoms need further description?

You tell Mr. C. that he needs to be on his back and assist him to that position. When you inspect his sheath site, you find that a 5 cm pool of blood has collected beneath the transparent dressing. His pedal pulses remain 2+ bilaterally. You place a 10 # sandbag over the site. You medicate Mr. C w/Sublimaze 50 mcg IV.

2. Write a follow-up narrative note.

3. What data must be included regarding the medication?

Case Study 7.5a

1030: Mrs. A, an 86-year-old female, has returned to the ICU post colectomy. You are the receiving RN. The anesthesiologist provides the following information: she was stable throughout a total colectomy for cancer; her estimated blood loss was 1000 cc; she received 2500 cc LR during the case; she is allergic to sulfa; she has an epidural catheter with Fentanyl and Marcaine at 4 cc/hr.

1030: Your initial assessment is lethargic w/ mumbling, incoherent speech, opens eyes slowly to noxious stimuli, MAE (moves all extremities) weakly to pain, not following commands; HR 68, R 10, BP 110/40, T 35.8°C; O_2 sat 96% on 50% face mask. Her dressing covers her entire abdomen, which is large, firm and distended. There are 2 wound drains connected to Hemovac suction. Her IV is LR at 200 cc/hr. She has a urinary catheter to drainage. She has a nasal gastric tube, which you connect to low suction.

1. Prioritize the objective and subjective data for written documentation.

    OBJECTIVE   SUBJECTIVE

    _____   _____
    _____   _____
    _____   _____
    _____   _____
    _____   _____
    _____   _____

2. Write a verbal report for presentation to the nursing instructor.

    _____
    _____
    _____

3. Write an admitting note.

    _____
    _____
    _____
    _____

Case Study 7.5b

1045: You remain at the bedside to closely monitor Mrs. A. You have covered her with warmed blankets. She is becoming more arousable, begins to moan when awake, and then drifts back to unconsciousness. When she is awake, she weakly reaches toward her face with her right arm. Her O_2 sat is 94%, HR 100, R14, BP 110/50.

1. Write a follow-up narrative note.

    _____
    _____
    _____
    _____

Case Study 7.5c

1100: Mrs. A is now awake and moaning continuously. She answers your questions in 2 and 3 word sentences. She restlessly tugs at her oxygen mask. Her O_2 sat is 98%. HR 110, R 22, BP 130/48. You ask if she is in pain. She nods her head and moans. You increase the rate of her epidural to 5 cc/hr and give her a bolus dose as well.

1115: Mrs. A. is quiet after the increase in analgesia. HR 90, R 16, BP 100/50, R 36.1°C. O_2 sat 99%. You change her oxygen to 6 L nasal cannula. You notice that it has been 1 hour since her arrival. You observe that her urinary output has been 20 cc for that hour. Her wound drains have collected a total of 200 cc bloody drainage. Her abdominal dressing is clean, dry, and intact. Her NG is draining tan.

1. Write a follow-up narrative note.

_____

_____

_____

_____

_____

Case Study 7.6

You are assigned to attend rounds with a home care nurse. The first patient is Mrs. K, a 77-year-old widowed white female. She lives alone in quiet middle class neighborhood and has two sons, both living over 200 miles away. She is regularly visited by the home health nurse for ocular problems. Her ocular history includes:

Drug-induced ocular cicatricial pemphigoid: chronic, progressive blistering and scarring of the mucous membranes of the eyes

Symblepharon: adhesions of palpebral conjunctiva to bulbar conjunctiva, glaucoma OU, severe, long standing, with history of poor compliance to medication regimen

Trichiasis: lashes turning in toward the eyeball

Distichiasis: double row of eyelashes

Entropion: turning in of eyelids

Legal blindness with visual acuity (VA): OD:CF (counts fingers) @ 2 feet; OS 20/400.

The visit on this day is to assess a foreign body sensation and excessive tearing in her left eye.

In preparing for the visit you read the past history specific to vision problems. The history includes:

Recurrent corneal erosion

Corneal ulcer OS

Pseudophakia OU

Pannus (corneal neovascularization) OS secondary to pemphigoid

Corneal scarring OS

Optic disc damage OD (.9 disc/cup ratio)

IOP (intraocular pressure) OU have been as high as 60 (normal IOP = 7−22)

Disc hemorrhage OD (secondary to long-standing glaucoma)

Retinal vein occlusion OD

Her ocular surgical history is status post:

Cyclophotocoagulation OD (decreasing aqueous productions)

Cataract surgery OU

Entropion repair $\bar{c}$ mucous membrane graft

Electrolysis/epilation OU: ongoing

You also review the general medical history for the patient in order to be prepared for assessment or treatment complications during the visit. The past general medical history includes the following:

Anemia

Osteoarthritis

GI hemorrhage (5 months ago)

Colostomy with mucous fistula (5 months ago)

Open abdominal wound

Right hip replacement (11 months ago)

Right knee replacement (10 months ago)

Hypothyroidism

Allergies: All preservatives

A note on her mental status reveals that Mrs. K is alert and oriented but has a history of anxiety and depression. The note states that she is often "overwhelmed and frustrated" with her multiple ocular problems, deteriorating vision, and progressive loss of independence.

She has been able to live independently without live-in care, eats a regular diet that she prepares herself, and maintains her medication schedule; however, home care nurses assist her in identifying her ophthalmic solutions and preparing and checking expiration dates of her oral medications.

Her medications are as follows (preservative-free medications are marked with an asterisk):

Timolol* .5% gtt 1 OU bid

Pilocarpine* 2% gtt 1 qid

Vitamin A* ophthalmic ung OU lids bid

Sulfacetamide* 10% gtt 1 OS qid (when bandage contact lens in place)

Artificial tears* prn

Diamox (acetazolamide) 125 mg po tid (hydration needs)

Thyroid 1 grs. QD

Tylenol XS 500 mg po prn

Naprosyn 250 mg po prn

Darvocet -N 100 po q 4 hr prn

Cytoxan - (Cyclophosphamide) (dc'd)

The most recent lab work in her chart included basic chemistry; electrolytes; liver function studies (LFS); lipids (cholesterol level 200–260) (triglycerides 200–201)

She is most concerned about her loss of independence. She is unable to identify her eye medications as they are all made up without preservatives and have frequent and different outdates. She does not fully understand, or is in denial of, her grave visual prognosis. She has knowledge deficit of medication use, purpose, and effects, particularly hydration needs while on carbonic anhydrase inhibitors (Diamox [acetazolamide]). She is at risk for kidney stone formation, fluid volume deficit, and electrolyte imbalance while on this drug.

She makes ophthalmologist visits 2–3 times per week for electrolysis or removal of turned-in lashes that are impinging on conjunctiva or cornea. Her ever-present fear is that of permanent vision loss. Occasional eye cultures have grown staphylococcus, and she has had several courses of Ciloxan ophthalmic solution for treatment of infection.

You realize that the ongoing problem with osteoarthritis also complicates her ability to properly administer her eye medications and increases the risk for poor compliance and inadequate control of intraocular pressure. Her anemia affects her energy level and alters her healing ability.

You arrive for your visit and find Mrs. K to be alert and exhibiting signs of anxiety. She is holding her magnifier in her shaking hands and states that she wishes she could see what is causing her eye to hurt. She speaks in short phrases, darting her head to address both you and the home care nurse. She is wiping around her left eye with a tissue.

You observe as the ophthalmic nurse carefully examines Mrs. K's eye, including fluorescein staining, and decides to remove several lashes that are impinging on the cornea. Fluorescein staining reveals no corneal erosion. The conjunctiva has minimal injection and the tearing is clear and without suspicious exudate. The ophthalmic RN monitors the IOP OU, which reveals IOPs of 20 and 18.

The ophthalmic nurse reviews the importance of punctal occlusion while coaching Mrs. K in the proper method of instillation of daily eye medications. The nurse checks the expiration dates on the eye solutions and writes out the dates in large bold print so Mrs. K can call and order a refill on a timely basis. Because some of the medications are preservative-free and require refrigeration, the nurse is able to inspect and determine if Mrs. K has unspoiled food available. The refrigerator appears well stocked and the dates on the milk and juice are current.

The nurse informs Mrs. K that the lashes impinging on her cornea were removed. She asks Mrs. K how her eye feels now and asks if she has any further questions or problems at this time. Mrs. K is now sitting, her hands folded. She speaks without extraneous head movement and states, "I am fine now; the scratchy feeling in my eye is gone and my eye pressures are the same as at the doctor's office last week."

Before you leave, Mrs. K is instructed to avoid rubbing her eyes, wipe any tears with clean tissues, and be sure to wash her hands frequently, particularly before and after instilling her eye medications. Mrs. K was reminded to take 8 oz. of water with her Diamox. Signs and symptoms to report to the MD are reviewed with Mrs. K, such as increased, unrelieved pain; foreign body sensation; sudden further loss of vision; and/or increased tearing.

1. Prioritize the objective and subjective data for written documentation of the current home visit.

   OBJECTIVE   SUBJECTIVE

   _____   _____

   _____   _____

   _____   _____

   _____   _____

   _____   _____

   _____   _____

   _____   _____

2. Write a problem-specific nursing note for this visit.

   Subjective:

   _____

   _____

   _____

   Objective:

   _____

   _____

   _____

Problem List

_____

_____

_____

_____

_____

_____

_____

_____

_____

_____

3. Write a personal social history.

_____

_____

_____

Case Study 7.7a

You are given a one-to-one assignment in the ICU. The assigned patient, Mr. L, is a 58-year-old stockbroker who has had recurrent episodes of abdominal pain and occult blood in his stool. His vital signs on admission were BP 100/60, P 92, R 18, T 98.6°F. You enter his room and notice that he appears pale. He has an NG tube in his left naris, which you assess to be patent; and the external features of the nose are clean with no redness or discharge. When asked he states that he does not feel nauseated. You note that he is very cooperative with her interview and is alert and oriented. He tells you that his daughter is a nurse and that he is comfortable being cared for by a student.

You do a head-to-toe physical and record that the patient is tachycardic but that the heart rate is regular. His skin is moist and cool and the nailbed capillary refill is slow at 4 seconds. Both lungs are clear to auscultation, without crackles, and he is receiving O_2 at 2 l/min through a nasal cannula. The pulse oximeter reads 99%. The abdominal assessment is normal with positive bowel sounds in all quadrants. You palpate gently and feels that the belly is soft and without any gross abnormalities. The patient states that the palpation causes him no discomfort. While you are in the room the patient asks to use the urinal. He is able to urinate 70 ml of dark amber urine. You remember that admitting urine specific gravity read 1.025. Before leaving the room you check the IV sites and note that there were two 16 g IVs, one in each arm; both were patent and infusing NS @ 75 cc/hr. He had received blood during the night shift and had a hematocrit of 28, which had been drawn on hour after the delivery of the first unit of packed red blood cells (PRBC).

1. Prioritize the objective and subjective data for written documentation.

OBJECTIVE	SUBJECTIVE
_____	_____
_____	_____
_____	_____
_____	_____
_____	_____
_____	_____

2. Write a verbal report for presentation to the nursing instructor.

_____

_____

_____

_____

3. Write an admitting note.

_____

_____

_____

_____

Case Study 7.7b

You review the nursing plan in the patient's chart, which shows that the patient received 3 liters of normal saline lavage through the NG tube along with the blood transfusion. When you next visit the patient at 0200, he states: "I feel cold."

You review all of the known data near the end of the clinical day and prioritize the following in determining NANDA diagnoses Mr. L:

1. Mr. L is demonstrating poor perfusion based on the nailbed refill and is undergoing fluid and blood replacement through two IV sites; a second unit of packed cells is ready for transfusion later in the day. His oxygen demand is being supplemented at 2 liters by nasal cannula. You know that checking vital signs at hourly intervals, assessing the patency of the IVs, and delivering the packed cells are essential interventions for establishing acceptable tissue perfusion. You choose a nursing diagnosis of "alteration in tissue perfusion—peripheral, related to hypovolemia."

2. You are also concerned about the patient's complaint of "feeling cold" and recognize the possible interventions as independent nursing function. You decide that providing warmed blankets and assessing the efficacy of this intervention every two hours are appropriate actions that should increase the patient's level of comfort as well as provide circulatory support. You include the NANDA diagnosis "alteration in comfort—related to temperature regulation" to the plan of care.

3. You choose to be proactive in Mr. L's care plan by recognizing the he is NPO with direct intravenous fluid replacement. Although he is hypovolemic, he is still at risk for fluid overload with possible pulmonary complications, such as edema, indicating frequent assessment of lung sounds. You decide to include the nursing diagnosis "potential for fluid volume overload" in the care plan.

Your assignment includes documenting according to the clinical unit's guidelines. The unit is currently using a SOAP format.

1. Write a note using the SOAP format.

Subjective:

_____

_____

_____

Objective:

_____

_____

_____

Assessment/Plan

_____

_____

_____

_____

_____

_____

_____

_____

_____

 Case Study 7.8a

Clara Reynolds arrives in the labor and delivery suite at 1000 holding her abdomen and saying, "Something is not right in my stomach." A brief interview reveals that Clara believes she is pregnant and has been experiencing low abdominal cramping the past 24 hours. The frequency and intensity of the cramps have escalated over the past six hours. Clara states, "It took a long time to get a ride here." She finally located a friend who escorted her to the L&D entrance.

The preadmission assessment reveals that Clara is an anxious, single, 17-year-old with suspected poor nutrition, skin dry and flaking, poor turgor, mucous membranes pale, BP 140/74, T 99°F, P 92, R 20. Abd. soft and pregnant, fundal height 26 cm, urine specimen concentrated: dipstick: pH 7, 4+ protein and large ketones. External fetal monitor applied per L&D protocol: FHR 160, uterine contractions q 4–8 min apart lasting 40–50 seconds, vaginal exam (V.E.) deferred, no obvious vaginal secretions. L&D on-call obstetrician notified of status and need for MD evaluation.

MD orders: initiate IV c̄ 1000 cc NS @ 150 cc/hr, draw blood specimen for CBC c̄ diff, type and hold clot and electrolytes. Straight cath for urine specimen, send to lab for U/A and microscopic exam.

1. Prioritize the objective and subjective data for written documentation.

   OBJECTIVE   SUBJECTIVE

   _____   _____

   _____   _____

   _____   _____

   _____   _____

   _____   _____

   _____   _____

   _____   _____

2. Write a verbal report for presentation to the nursing instructor.

   _____

   _____

   _____

   _____

3. Write an admitting note.

   _____

   _____

   _____

   _____

Case Study 7.8b

1200: Further findings reveal that Clara has been experiencing urinary frequency and urgency without dysuria for the past week. Yesterday she began to feel contractions and did not understand what was causing the abdominal pain. Clara, who does not have an identified health care provider, typically seeks treatment for specific health crises at the closest ER. She has not sought prenatal care for this pregnancy but states she was sure she was pregnant. LMP unknown, gravida 3 para 0. Clara reports two therapeutic abortions six months apart, the last was one year ago at local free clinic. Weight: 100 lbs., Height: 5′ 2,″ smokes less than 1 pack of cigarettes/day, denies using street or prescription drugs, denies any ETOH use. The father is unavailable.

Clara is emancipated from her family. However, one sister remains close and supportive. Also a neighbor is a good friend and usually available to assist. However, both are currently out of town.

IV initiated c̄ #18 angiocath at left dorsum hand. 1000 cc NS superimposed and infusing at 150 cc/hr. Serum specimen transported to lab for evaluation of CBC c̄ diff, type and hold clot and electrolytes. Straight cathed for urine specimen; dark amber color, cloudy c̄ particulate matter. Specimen sent to lab. for U/A and microscopic exam.

Physical exam performed by MD reveals: V.E.: long, thick, closed, and posterior.

Clara is admitted for further treatment for a suspected bladder infection. The plan includes: develop high risk plan of care and notify social services for discharge planning.

1. Write a follow-up note.

   _____

   _____

   _____

   _____

2. What would you add to CHH?

   _____

   _____

   _____

   _____

Case Study 7.9a

You are taking an admitting history. Your patient is a 15-year-old female whose mother "dropped" her off at the emergency room and who is complaining of abdominal pain and vaginal cramping. Preliminary admitting diagnosis is urinary tract infection. She weighs 75 kg and has no known drug allergies. Vital signs are T 36°C po, P 105, R 20, BP 152/85.

Her past history includes Type II diabetes treated with oral glipizide 10 mg twice a day, with an admitting FSBS of 350. She has also been diagnosed with asthma (RAD) and was prescribed an inhaler, Vanceril, 2 puffs q6 prn. She also takes Vicodin 1 tab qd for "pain." She uses her mom's pain pills.

She volunteers the following information: "My bladder hurts every time I pee," and continues to have back pain and cramping. Her last normal menstrual period (LNMP) was 12/98. She has had no follow-up in the endocrine clinic related to her diabetes. However, she says that "My twin put me on insulin because the pills weren't working and she decides my sliding scale."

She shares her schedule with you: FSBS [finger stick blood sugar] is usually 200–300.

Sliding scale as determined by her sibling:

>95 5u reg

>200 15 u

>300 25 u

She is admitted for admit for candidal vaginitis & DM management. The hospital social worker contacts her mother who responds, "Yeah, I know she is taking my insulin. I have diabetes and I know how much to give her." A CPS [Child Protective Services] referral is made, and the mother replied "Oh Lordy, not again."

1. Prioritize the objective and subjective data for written documentation.

    OBJECTIVE   SUBJECTIVE

    _____   _____

    _____   _____

    _____   _____

    _____   _____

    _____   _____

    _____   _____

2. Write a verbal report for presentation to the nursing instructor.

    ____ _____

    _____

    _____

    _____

3. Write an admitting note.

    _____

    _____

    _____

    _____

Case Study 7.9b

You are assigned to complete CHH and ROS. The teen's affect is quiet and friendly. Her general appearance is appropriate for age and she is cooperative during the interview. She appears depressed, looking out the window and speaking only when spoken to. She does not smile and answers appropriately but offers no information beyond the exact question.

When asked, she states she lives with her mom who is a diabetic and who recently had a below-the-knee amputation of her right leg (BKA R) and her twin sister who is also DM Type II, and 2 brothers. Her dad lives in the area and has only peripheral involvement with her.

Her extended family is not supportive but she displays an uncharacteristic smile response when she talks about the support of her boyfriend. She attends a continuation high school, which is run by a religious organization; she states she "likes school." She reads at the third grade level, but states she wants "to go to college and make something of myself."

Her mom is aware of the twins' insulin use and refused to bring them to consult with an MD for diabetic control and teaching. The patient reports "I beg my mother to take me to the doctor."

P/S & sexual hx: With downcast eyes she responds quietly that 6 mo. ago she was "kidnapped, beaten, raped, and left by an unknown male assailant, which was reported to the police." She says "I still have flashbacks" and "Mom would never take me for counseling and she tells me all the time it was my fault and I deserved it." She has a negative past hx for STDs, negative for drug and ETOH use, and she states that "people think it's cool but it's not." Her history is positive for suicide attempt with a razor blade and ideation 2 months ago which was aborted by her boyfriend. No other attempts were acknowledged.

The student noted on the next clinical day that the teen placed a self-imposed police hold on herself when ready for discharge to home because of a history of child abuse and neglect, as well as medical neglect. She states: "I love my mom but I think I should have more help with this since I am only 15. I would rather go to a foster family." She "doesn't feel safe with her mother and her mom hits her with fists repeatedly on daily basis." There is a history of verbal abuse, and the teen discloses that her mom could "write a dictionary on cuss words because she uses them all." She was awaiting foster placement as no place was available for someone her age.

She is finally discharged 2 weeks post admit to group foster home, awaiting single family placement. There is an ongoing CPS intervention regarding the teen and other siblings. Discharge orders include:

Doxy 100 mg bid times ten days

insulin sliding scale

15 u nph

nph bid

glipizide po bid

Cont Vanceril as before

Follow-up c̄ teen clinic, rape counseling

1. Write a discharge note for this patient.

_____
_____
_____
_____

2. Write the following additional data for the CHH.

   General Appearance

_____
_____
_____
_____

   Family History

_____
_____
_____
_____

   Personal/Social and Sexual History

_____
_____
_____
_____
_____
_____

Case Study 7.10a

You are assigned a 2 1/2-year-old boy who was admitted for I & D (incision and drainage) L calcaneus secondary to 4 wk hx osteomyelitis L heel.

He first presented to the ER when his parents noticed that the child was having difficulty walking and then began limping over the course of two weeks. Lab work and X-rays were negative, and he was discharged to home with instructions "to watch him" and that problem would "resolve on its own."

The parents noticed in the following week that there was no improvement and has in fact worsened. His L heel is slightly swollen and reddened. They returned to the ER, which resulted in a repeat of negative findings. He was discharged with no change in instructions.

Three days after the second ER visit the mother of the baby (MOB) noticed that the toddler was "crawling only," and presented at the orthopedic clinic where the child's previous X-rays were reviewed and a second series of X-rays were taken. There appeared to be a hairline fracture and a cast was placed on the L foot for 2 weeks. When cast was removed, the L heel was noted to be swollen, reddened, tender, and hot to touch. A decision was made to proceed with I & D L heel based on symptoms consistent with osteomyelitis.

The preanesthesia assessment showed:

URI [upper respiratory infection] s/p [status post] 2 wks

Probable osteomyelitis × 4 wks L heel

Weight 13.8 kg

BP 122/69, P 128, R 24, T 36.5°C axillary. NPO solids/milk, Motrin 200 prn pain q6. NKDA. General anesthesia planned for I & D and percutaneous line placement in OR.

The surgery was uneventful. The surgery was recorded as an "I & D of the L calcaneus with drain placement and casting of the L foot with a cast 'window' over wound." A #3 French percutaneous line with a beveled end was placed in the L AC (anterior cubital) (61 cm cath, 11 cm in, 50 cm out) while the child was under anesthesia (with 2 failed attempts R AC) with minimal blood loss. The line was flushed with 100 u heparin/cc 3 cc without resistance.

The PNP (pediatric nurse practitioner) was called to PAR (postanesthesia recovery) when oozing blood was noted at the perc line insertion site. Direct pressure was applied for 15 min. and the bleeding controlled. EBL was < 3 cc, the dressing changed and pressure tape applied. A later assessment revealed "some swelling to the fingers"; however, the line flushed with no resistance.

1. Prioritize the objective and subjective data for written documentation.

   OBJECTIVE   SUBJECTIVE

   _____   _____
   _____   _____
   _____   _____
   _____   _____
   _____   _____
   _____   _____
   _____   _____

2. Write a verbal report for presentation to the nursing instructor.

   _____
   _____
   _____

Case Study 7.10b

Postop assessment of the foot and heel revealed CMS L foot WNL. The patient is brought to the floor with the following orders: LLE elevation, CMS checks q 2–4 c̄ TPR checks, Motrin 200 mg q 6 prn pain, Tylenol 200 mg po q 4–6 prn pain. Tylenol codeine elixir 5 cc q 3 RTC, MSo4 1 mg IV q 1 hr prn severe pain, Kefzol 500 mg q 8 IV, L hand PIV hep locked c̄ 10 u cc 2 ccs q 4–6 hrs and prn, D5 1/3 NS 10 KCL/500 cc IV @ 40 cc/hr until taking po well. CBC & ESR with AM draw.

When you arrive the nursing notes read:

0800 T 37.1°C ax, HR 144, R 30, BP 140/80, ESR 92, CRP 3.2, cultures pending, labs elevated. Pos. CMS L ft. Kefzol due @ 0900. Crying with approach of med personnel. Perc line infusing @ 40 cc/hr. Site feels swollen but soft, IV pump infusing s̄ alarms/occlusions. CMS to fingers good. Taking minimal PO's. Voiding well in diaper. Parents at bedside. Mom states "He's starting to get fussy. It's about time for his pain med." Tyco elixir given po as scheduled.

0900: Relief from pain noted. Asleep, resting comfortably. Kefzol infusing s̄ difficulty via perc line.

1000: MD ortho clinician in to see pt, no significant findings.

You assess the R arm, which appears swollen, and you believe the perc line may be infiltrated. You consult with the staff RN, who has "never seen a perc line infiltrate" and does not suspect that could be the problem. The R arm is assessed and is swollen, tight, and red extending to the upper arm. You remove the child's gown and observe the swelling is from the shoulder/upper chest area to below the nipple line on the right arm. Dependent edema is assessed lateral and posterior to the R shoulder blade. (You feel like an idiot for not lifting the gown earlier.) You immediately discontinue the R AC perc line and note that the beveled tip is intact. The catheter measures 61 cm tip to end. The crying and fussiness is attributed to 24 hr postop status for I & D. The MD is notified as there is concern about possible compartment syndrome. Warm compresses are applied every hour for the next 16 hrs with frequent arm assessments. The staff believes that the line was never properly placed. The parents are educated about the course of care and support for them is prioritized.

1. Write a follow-up narrative note.

_____

_____

_____

Case Study 7.10c

At noon after warm compresses have been applied the child is less irritable and resting quietly when not disturbed. He is eating small amounts of food without difficulty. He continues to run a fever of 100.3°F, and the culture comes back positive for a rare staph C negative infection. This result is considered possible but unlikely, and antibiotics are continued as ordered.

1. Write an follow-up narrative note.

_____

_____

_____

Case Study 7.10d

Four hours later there is a noticeable decrease in swelling of the left arm and the child is raising the arm and reaching for his toys. He is afebrile, T 98.8°F, is eating regular food, and is laughing and playing in his bed. His peripheral IV is patent. Tylenol is given to control pain. The nurse continues to apply warm compresses.

1. Write a follow-up narrative note.

_____

_____

_____

BOX 7.1

Review of Systems

A. General status: perception of health, weight/weight changes, weakness, fatigue, fever, chills, dizziness, sweating (diaphoresis), anorexia, malaise

B. Skin, hair, nails: color/color changes, texture, pruritis (itching), growth, care, tone, rashes, lumps, dryness, change in pigmented areas, bruising (ecchymosis, petechia with age dating), bleeding

C. Eyes: diplopia, itching, burning, visual disturbance, inflammation (redness), lacrimation (excessive), glasses/contacts/IOL, cataracts, glaucoma, sclera, AC depth, IOP, hyphema, visual acuity, halos, photophobia, color blindness, night blindness, pain, discharge

D. Ears: hearing changes, tinnitus, vertigo, pain, OM, excess cerumen, vertigo, external, internal, position, equality, discharge, infection, itching

Situation

Patient complains that *your* voice sounds muffled.

Assessment/observation: Ear assessment shows large amount of earwax preventing you from seeing the tympanic membrane.

Documentation: c/o hearing decreased, T/M obscured, lg amt cerumen, otoscope exam or unable to visualize TM due to cerumen obstruction

E. Nose, sinus: congestion (stuffiness), discomfort, epistaxis (nosebleeds), discharge, symmetry

F. Mouth, throat: bleeding, sores, color, dental care, dentes, hygiene, flossing, dysphagia, pain, hoarseness, URI, ROM, halitosis, lumps, glands goiter

G. Breasts: pain, discharge, nipple change, BSE, lumps, symmetry/asymmetry, dimpling, trauma, swelling

H. Respiratory: asthma, cough, dyspnea, orthopnea, PND, hemoptysis, sleep position & pattern, number of pillows, wheezing, crackles, bronchitis, sputum, exposures (TB, occupational), smoking (pack history)

I. Cardiovascular: murmur, arrhythmia, pain, varicosities, phlebitis, HTN, palpitations, apnea, orthopnea, dyspnea (with/without exertion), paroxysmal dyspnea, cyanosis, peripheral edema

J. Gastrointestinal: appetite, N, V, D, constipation, BM pattern, GERD, heartburn, BRBPR (bright red blood per rectum), jaundice, dysphagia, bloating (gas), hematemesis, food intolerance, belching, rectal bleeding, abdominal pain (quadrants), hematochezia, black tarry stools

K. Urinary tract: pain, hesitancy, urgency, frequency, burning, color, stones, hematuria, incontinence, discharge, force of stream, dysuria, polyuria, nocturia

L. Genital: TSE, discharge, dyspareunia, lesions, STD, changes, menses (onset, last, regularity, breakthrough, length, amount), GPSABTAB, sexual function, practices, difficulties, itching

M. Musculoskeletal: pain, swelling, stiffness, sprains, congenital deformity, ROM

N. Neuro: syncope, vertigo, dizziness, tingling, numbness, muscle weakness, gait, speech, balance

O. Endocrine: polydipsia, polyphagia, polyuria, heat/cold intolerance, irritability, hair loss, wt. change

P. Hematopoietic: bruising, bleeding, gingivitis

Q. Psychological status: mood swings, apathy, suicidal ideation, change in appetite, change in sex drive, wt. change, concentration, irritability, memory disturbance, preoccupation

R. OB/GYN: age of menarche, P, G, SAB, TAB, LMP, LNMP, reg/irreg, Pap smear, mammography, BSE, sexual activity, urinary incontinence, menopause, STD, contraception

Case Study 7.10e

0800: T 37.9°C ax, HR 104, R 24, BP 108/68. Arm almost return to normal. Good ROM, CMS R fingers & arm. Arm bends easily. Slept well per parents. Plain ty 1 time noc. PIV infusing, hep lock p̄ 0900 abx to playroom, TV Cont abx

0900: MSo4 2 mg by ortho prior to drain removal. Good effect. Smiling, laughing, states, "My arm doesn't hurt anymore," swinging arm and giggling.

0930: Drain pulled c̄ sm amt blood loss, no distress. Repeat culture rare staph C neg. Probable discharge to home post arm assessment & ed on home IV therapy.

1600: Stable , VSS, afebrile, playing, laughing, fluid resorbed R arm, 0 ROM limitations R arm, CMS L toes, R fingers WNL. DC to home c̄ IV abx, home health referral, f/u RTC 2 days.

1. Write a discharge note.

_____

_____

_____

_____

_____

_____

_____

BOX 7.2

Value Added: Good Interviewing Yields Critical Data

One morning in the late 1970s, on a very active postpartum unit, a typical day shift was taking shape. Staff, with assignments in hand, began the routines that would accomplish patient care needs.

Preparations for multiple patient discharges were well under way. Back then we used a very primitive form of discharge planning, consisting of an exit interview and a physical assessment. Both pieces of information were recorded on a checklist. One of the questions we asked related to what type of birth control was planned.

During one specific interview the birth control information was queried. The mother's response was, "Well, I guess the diaphragm is not effective for me." Further conversation regarding why this particular method was precluded revealed that this was the fourth unplanned pregnancy for this midthirties, university-educated woman. Dredging deeper into the facts of diaphragm use, the woman disclosed some very interesting facts.

She indicated that she was told "any type of jelly could be used with the diaphragm when inserting it." Very matter of factly she responded, "With all these children there is always grape jelly in the cabinet." Subsequent dialogue about placement of the device all seemed appropriate: inserted before intercourse, was able to palpate cervix approximately in the center of the ring, left it in for 12 hours after an intimate experience. Our conversation continued, the woman indicated after purchasing her diaphragm from the pharmacy and upon returning home she would remove the bladder or bowl from the device. She did so because when she was measured for and instructed on use of the diaphragm at the clinic there was not a bladder on the ring. She thought that it was superfluous material.

This anecdote demonstrates the importance of appropriate follow-up interview and documentation. The nurses did not assume that the patient had received accurate information regarding the use of her diaphragm for birth control. Nor was there the assumption that because the patient was well educated she would necessarily have the necessary health care information. The nurse intuitively reviewed the facts involving the failure of the diaphragm to prevent pregnancy, set aside class bias, and provided good health education for her patient.

Answer Guide

Exercise 7.1

1. tremors
   Common: trembling as in slight earth shaking
   Technical: body movement that is involuntary, usually a slight tremble can be regular or intermittent

2. output
   Common: amount of work, energy, or product produced within a time frame
   Technical: quantity of urine, excretion, or other measured substance over a given period

3. fixation
   Common: strong attachment or obsession
   Technical: being immobilized and firmly attached; preserving tissue sample for analysis

4. stream
   Common: body of water running in channel of earth's surface
   Technical: steady flow of liquid, especially urine

5. intake
   Common: a taking in; place in a pipe where water is taken in
   Technical: amount of food or fluid absorbed by patient

6. block
   Common: solid section of wood usually with flat sides; section of a city with defined parameters
   Technical: interruption in the transmission of impulse, e.g., cardiac or nerve

7. expire
   Common: come to an end; to die
   Technical: breathe out; to die

8. relief
   Common: lessening of discomfort; aid given to needy; art or map with elevated components
   Technical: alleviation of symptom; area under prosthesis intended to reduce pressure

9. reduce
   Common: lessen or diminish
   Technical: restore by manipulation or surgery to normal position

10. trigger
    Common: a release for discharging a firearm
    Technical: a stimulus for a physiological or chemical event

Case Study 7.1a

1. Prioritize the objective and subjective data for written documentation.

OBJECTIVE	SUBJECTIVE
75 y/o	"not sick"
F	severe "stomach" pain
widow	"doubled up"
10-year hx diverticulitis	"constipation"
"trickle" BM	loud BS
liquids only × 3 days	embarrassment
Bactrim from Mexico	
X-ray	

2. Using the CHH format, record known data as you would in a patient record.
   First admission for Mrs. F, 75 y/o, F, widow, lives alone, c/o "severe stomach pain" causing her to "double up," "constipation" c̄ loud "gurgling sounds," does not "feel sick," BM "trickle," liquids only tolerated × 3 days, PH diverticulitis × 10 yr., self-administers Bactrim from Mexico, abd. X-ray inclusive, endoscopy reveals bowel obstruction, P/SH lives alone, embarrassed by BS.

3. List the data that are relevant and should be prioritized in history gathering.
   Onset and duration of the problem, pain assessment, Bactrim use and past effectiveness, past health history, nutrition history

4. Which key concepts are represented in your answer?
   Characteristics of symptom
   Subjective and objective information
   Format
   Spelling and handwriting
   Language application impact

Case Study 7.1b

1. What data would you consider in choosing the nursing diagnosis "Knowledge deficit related to health maintenance and disease prevention"?
   General good health, no health maintenance, 55 pack years, hx of ETOH

2. What key concepts might be useful in assessing health maintenance problems?
   Bias and judgmental issues regarding smoking and alcohol use

3. What data would you consider in choosing the nursing diagnosis "Knowledge deficit r/t effective management of diverticulitis"?
   Possible surgery, possible colostomy, hx of self treatment

Case Study 7.1c

1. With the available data, write an objective discharge assessment that describes Mrs. F's adjustment to the colostomy.
   temporary colostomy, "this thing," states acceptance, good eye contact, go home, states pain only c̄ movement & cough, VS stable, goal "take down," help available, d/c to home care.

Case Study 7.2a

1. Prioritize the objective and subjective data for written documentation.

OBJECTIVE	SUBJECTIVE
55 y/o	"difficulty breathing"
M	restless
VS T 98.6°F, HR 100, BP 140/80, R 20.	slightly diaphoretic
Pulse ox = 90%	no pallor
OTC antihistamines	unable to "catch breath"
no allergy meds × 30 years	
X-ray no infiltrates	
bronchial wheezes > c̄ forced expiration	
neg smoking hx	
neg hx CAD	
pos hx "hay fever"	
neg chest pain	
SOBOE	

2. Write a verbal report for presentation to the nursing instructor.
   Mr. D is a 55-year-old male who presents to ER with complaint of "difficulty breathing," vital signs are BP 140/80, HR 120, R 30, T 98.6°F, O₂ sat 90%, negative for chest pain, positive for restlessness, mild diaphoresis, bronchial

wheeze greater with forced expiration, chest X-ray is normal, past history of "hay fever" relieved by over the counter antihistamines. Treatment includes O_2 2 l/m per nasal cannula, head at 45°, and bronchodilator; skin pink O_2 sat 95%, admitted for further evaluation.

3. Write an admitting note using CHH format.
   Mr. D, 55 y/o M to ER, c/o "difficulty breathing," VS BP 140/80, HR 120, R 30, T 98.6, O_2 sat 90%, − chest pain, + restlessness, mildly diaphoretic, bronchial wheeze > with forced expiration, CXR wnl, PH: "hay fever" relieved by OTC antihistamines. Tx: O_2 2 l/m per nasal cannula, head at 45°, bronchodilator. Admit for eval, d'c from ER skin pink, O_2 sat 95%.

Case Study 7.2b

1. State the objective findings that you include in the end of shift documentation.
   position
   pulse ox 98%
   skin warm, dry
   NBCF sec
   neg for sob ambulating
   neg wheeze on forced exp
   lungs clear
   HR 80
   R 20

2. Write a verbal report for presentation to the nursing instructor.
   Mr. D 55 y/o M, 1 day post-admit respiratory dysfunction, NAD [no acute distress], HR 80, R 20, lung fields clear, O_2 sat 98, negative for wheeze, no shortness of breath ambulating.

Case Study 7.2c

1. Write a discharge note.
   Mr. D, 55 y/o M, d'c to home, HR 80, R 20, lung fields clear, O_2 sat 98%, − wheeze, SOBOE, c̄ d'c instruction: follow physician's instructions, RTC × 1 week, or immediately c̄ ↑ sx, record activities if sx repeat. Pt able to repeat back instructions.

Case Study 7.3a

1. Prioritize the objective and subjective data for written documentation.

OBJECTIVE	SUBJECTIVE
17 y/o	lethargic
F	P/SH boyfriend treats Ms. T "really well."

   hx of overdose × 2
   lives w/ mother
   VS P 80, R 12, BP 100/50
   arousable
   oriented × 3
   empty bottle of Tylenol on the floor
   1 g activated charcoal lavage per NG
   NG removed

2. Write a verbal report for presentation to the nursing instructor.
   Ms. T, 17 y/o, F, admit ICU2, diagnosis acetaminophen overdose, VS P 80, R 12, BP 100/50, lethargic but arousable, otherwise oriented × 3, treated in the ER with 1 g activated charcoal lavage per NG, which was subsequently removed. Past history of overdose × 2, P/SH raised by single mom, has a boyfriend whom mom says treats teen "very well."

3. Write an admitting note using CHH format.
   ID: Ms. T, 17 y/o F
   HPI: to ER via ambulance, admit to ICU2, dx acetaminophen OD. VS: P 80, R 12, BP 100/50, lethargic but arousable, otherwise O × 3, found by mother "on the living room couch, unarousable, with an empty bottle of Tylenol on the floor next to her."
   Tx: 1 g activated charcoal lavage per NG, which was subsequently removed.
   P Hx: OD × 2
   P/SH: lives c̄ mother, who is single, has boyfriend who treats Ms. T "really well."

Case Study 7.3b

1. Write a follow-up narrative for the chart.
   1800: VS T 37.4°F, P 60, R 14, BP 90/50, IV D5.45% NS infusing @ 100 cc/h, easily arousable to name, answers appropriately, speech clear & coherent, PERRLA, MAE, neg unilateral weakness, nausea, open wounds, visible scars, ROS: tongue midline, c̄ black discoloration, LNMP × 3 wks, NKDA.

Case Study 7.4a

1. Prioritize the objective and subjective data for written documentation.

OBJECTIVE	SUBJECTIVE
58 y/o	drowsy
M	pleasant
EKG sinus rhythm	no visible distress
7 French arterial sheath, R groin	"feels fine"
site, soft s̄ drainage	needs to keep his right leg straight
pedal pulses, 2+ bil	
HR 80, R 14, BP 136/70	
IV of NS @ 100 cc/hr	
lung sounds clear bilaterally	

2. Write a verbal report for presentation to the nursing instructor.
   Mr. C, 58 y/o, 2 hours status post cardiac catheterization, in no acute distress, drowsy, states that he "feels fine." EKG reads normal sinus rhythm. He has a 7 French arterial sheath in his right groin. The sheath site is soft and without drainage. Pedal pulses are 2+ bilaterally. VS: HR 80, R 14, BP 136/70. He has an IV of NS at 100 cc/hr. His lung sounds are clear bilaterally. Importance of lying supine and keeping his right leg straight explained.

3. Write an admitting note.
   58 y/o, M, 2 hr. s/p cardiac catheterization, NAD, drowsy, states he "feels fine," EKG NSR, 7 Fr arterial sheath R groin, site soft s̄ drainage, pedal pulses 2+ bil, HR 80, R 14, BP 136/70, IV of NS @ 100 cc/hr., lung sounds clear bil, supine c̄ R leg straight, importance of position explained.

Case Study 7.4b

1. What subjective symptoms need further description?
   "My back was really hurting."
   "Being on my side helps."
   "I kind of feel like I am urinating, though."

2. Write a follow-up narrative note.
   1700: c/o "back pain," sensation to urinate, 5 cm blood beneath drsg, pedal pulses 2+ bil, 10 # sandbag positioned on site, pt reminded to remain supine, medicated.

3. What data must be included regarding the medication?
   Medication, Dose, Route, Evaluation

Case Study 7.5a

1. Prioritize the objective and subjective data for written documentation.

OBJECTIVE	SUBJECTIVE
86 y/o	EBL [estimated blood loss] 1000 cc
F	stable
2500 cc LR fluid input	lethargic
allergy sulfa	mumbling, incoherent speech
epidural catheter w/ Fentanyl & Marcaine at 4 cc/hr.	MAE [moves all extremities] weakly to pain
HR 68, R 10, BP 110/40, T 35.8°C	neg following commands
O_2 sat 96% on 50% face mask	abdomen is large, firm, and distended
2 wound drains Hemovac suction	opens eyes slowly to noxious stimuli
IV is LR at 200 cc/hr	
urinary catheter to drainage	
nasal gastric tube, connect to low suction	
dressing covers her entire abdomen	

2. Write a verbal report for presentation to the nursing instructor.
   Mrs. A, 86 y/o F, admit to ICU post total colectomy, EBL 1000 cc, stable, IV fluids: 2500 cc LR, epidural catheter in place c̄ Fentanyl & Marcaine at 4 cc/hr., allergic to sulfa, assessment postop T 35.8°C, HR 68, R 10, BP 110/40, O_2 sat 96% on 50% face mask, lethargic, mumbling, incoherent speech, opens eyes slowly to noxious stimuli, moves all extremities, abdomen, large, firm and distended, covered by dressing, 2 Hemovac drains, IV LR @ 200 cc/hr, urinary catheter, NG to low suction.

3. Write an admitting note.
   ID: Mrs. A, 86 y/o, F
   Dx: post colectomy, Ca
   Anesthesia report: stable, total colectomy for Ca, EBL 1000 cc, IV fluids: 2500 cc LR, epidural catheter in place c̄ Fentanyl & Marcaine at 4 cc/hr.
   Allergy: sulfa

Case Study 7.5b

1. Write a follow-up narrative note.
   1045: ↑ arousal, moaning when awake, in & out of consciousness, purposeful movement reaches to face with R arm when awake, O_2 sat 94%, HR 100, R 14, BP 110/50, applied warm blankets

Case Study 7.5c

1. Write a follow-up narrative note.
   1100: Awake, moaning continuously, answers in 2 and 3 word sentences, tugs oxygen mask, O_2 sat is 98%, HR 110, R 22, BP 130/48, c/o pain, medicated c̄ bolus, ↑ epidural to 5 cc/hr.
   1115: quiet, T 36.1°C, HR 90, R 16, BP 100/50, O_2 sat 99%, O_2 6 L nasal cannula, UO 20 cc, 200 cc bloody drg, abd drsg clean, dry, intact, NG drg tan.

Case Study 7.6

1. Prioritize the objective and subjective data for written documentation.

OBJECTIVE	SUBJECTIVE
foreign body sensation	family out of area
excessive tearing	mental status: alert, oriented,
legally blind	anxious, depressed, overwhelmed, frustrated

2. Write a problem-specific nursing note for this visit.
   Subjective: Foreign body sensation and excessive tearing OS

Objective: Eyes: OS, lashes impinging on cornea, − erosion,
+ excessive clear tears, minimal conjunctival injection
P/SH: S/S anxiety, hand shaking, head darting, disrupted speech pattern
Problem List
Problem #1 Trichiasis corneal irritation
Assessment: external eye exam, corneal staining
Treatment: Lash removal
Problem #2 Anxiety r/t ocular discomfort
Treatment: S/A
Problem #3 Anxiety r/t maintaining independence
Treatment: S/A
Problem #4 Unstable IOP, knowledge deficit in proper method of instillation
Assessment: tonometry, medication inspection
Treatment: instruct in punctal occlusion, coaching in method of instillation
Problem # 5 knowledge deficit in hydration needs
Assessment: Inquire about intake and output, S/S of frequency or pain with
urination
Treatment: instruct in adequate hydration such as to take 8 oz. of water with
Diamox

3. Write a personal social history.
P/SH: Mrs. K, 78 y/o, widow $\bar{c}$ two sons, lives alone, single family residence,
family out of the area. Independence maintained though visual impairment
requires regular home health visits. History of anxiety and depression likely
r/t homebound status due to vision loss, decreased mobility, and ongoing
health problems.

Case Study 7.7a

1. Prioritize the objective and subjective data for written documentation.

OBJECTIVE	SUBJECTIVE
58 y/o	recurrent abdominal pain
M	appears pale
stockbroker	nose clean, no redness or discharge
+ occult blood in stool.	cooperative
BP 100/60, P 92, R 18, T 98.6°F	alert and oriented
NG tube left naris patent	skin is moist and cool
HRR, tachycardic	abdomen soft $\bar{s}$ gross abnormalities
Lungs clear bil., no crackles	no discomfort $\bar{c}$ palpation
NBCR 4 sec	
O_2 at 2 l/min per cannula	
O_2 sat 99%	
+BS all quadrants	
70 ml dark amber urine	
urine sg 1.025	
16 g IVs bil., patent, infusing NS @ 75 cc/hr	
one unit PRBC noc	
Hematocrit of 28	

2. Write a verbal report for presentation to the nursing instructor.
Cooperative 58 y/o M admit to ICU, diagnosis duodenal ulcer, VS: BP 100/60,
P 92, R 18, T 98.6°F, alert and oriented × 3, skin pale, moist and cool; cap refill
4 sec, lung fields clear bilateral, $\bar{s}$ crackles, O_2 at 2 l/min via nasal cannula, O_2
sat 99%, positive BS × 4 quadrants, urine dark amber with specific gravity of
1.025, 16 g IVs bil. patent and each infusing NS @ 75 cc/hr., Hct is 28 status
post one unit PRBCs, NG and IV sites intact, without redness.

3. Write an admitting note.
   58 y/o M admit to ICU, Dx duodenal ulcer, VS: BP 100/60, P 92, R 18, T 98.6°F, A & O × 3, cooperative, skin pale, moist & cool; cap refill (or NBCR) 4 sec, lung fields clear bil., neg crackles, O_2: 2 l/min via nasal cannula, O_2 sat 99%, + BS × 4, urine dark amber, sg 1.025, 16 g IVs bil. patent, infusing NS @ 75 cc/hr, Hct 28 status post one unit PRBC, NG & IV sites intact, s̄ redness.

Case Study 7.7b

1. Write a note using the SOAP format.
   Subjective: "foreign body sensation and excessive tearing OS"
   Objective: Eyes: OS, lashes impinging on cornea, − erosion, +excessive clear tears, minimal conjunctival injection

   Assessment/Plan

   1. A: alteration in tissue perfusion—peripheral, r/t hypovolemia
      P: • Check vital signs q 1°
         • Maintain IV patency
         • Transfuse second unit PRBC per order
         • Maintain O2 at 2 liters nasal cannula

   2. A: alteration in comfort—r/t temperature regulation
      P: • Provide warm blankets for comfort
         • Assess comfort level q 2° & prn

   3. A: potential for fluid volume overload
      P: • Maintain NPO status
         • Auscultate lung sounds for evidence of pulmonary edema q 2–4°
         • Notify physician of any Δ

Case Study 7.8a

1. Prioritize the objective and subjective data for written documentation.

OBJECTIVE	SUBJECTIVE
17 y/o	"Something is not right in my stomach."
F	urine concentrated
single	anxious
T 99°F, P 92, R 20, BP 140/74	poor nutrition
dry, flaking skin	low abd. cramping
poor turgor	
pale mucous membranes	
abd. soft, pregnant	
fundus 26 cm	
urine dipstick pH 7, + protein, + lg ketones	
FHR 160	
contractions q 4–8 min, 40–50 sec	
Neg vag d'c	

2. Write a verbal report for presentation to the nursing instructor.
   17 y/o, single, F presented to Labor and Delivery with complaint of "something is not right in my stomach," suspected pregnancy c̄ low abdominal cramping × 24 hours c̄ increasing frequency and intensity. VS BP 140/74, T 99°F, P 92, R 20, general appearance anxious, suspected poor nutrition, skin dry and flaking, poor turgor, mucous membranes pale, abd. soft, pregnant, fundal height 26 cm, urine concentrated. Dipstick: pH 7, 4+ protein, large ketones. External fetal monitor c̄ FHR 160, uterine contractions every 4–8 min lasting 40–50 seconds. V.E. deferred, no obvious vaginal secretions. On-call obstetrician notified of status and need for MD evaluation.

3. Write an admitting note.

   1100: 17 y/o, single, F, admit to L & D c/o "something is not right in my stomach," suspected pregnancy c̄ low abd. cramping × 24 hrs c̄ ↑ frequency, intensity, VS: BP 140/74, T 99°F, P 92, R 20.

   GA [general appearance]: anxious, suspected poor nutrition, skin dry and flaking, poor turgor, mucous membranes pale, abd. soft, pregnant, fundal ht 26 cm, FHR 160 ext monitor, uterine contractions every 4–8 min. lasting 40–50 sec., urine dipstick pH 7, 4+ protein, large ketones, VE deferred, no obvious vag secretions. O/C [on call] OB notified of status and need for evaluation.

Case Study 7.8b

1. Write a follow-up note.

   1200: c/o urinary frequency, urgency s̄ dysuria × week, onset of contractions 24 hrs, c̄ abd. pain, LMP unk , G3, P0, TAB2, IV c̄ #18 angiocath, L dorsum hand 1000 cc NS @ 150 cc/hr., CBC c̄ diff, type, hold clot, electrolytes to lab, straight cath urine spec dark amber, cloudy c̄ particulate to lab U/A and microscopic.

2. What would you add to CHH?

   GA: Wt: 100 lbs., Ht: 5′ 2″
   PMH: No primary provider, LMP unk, G3, P0, TAB2
   P/SH: emancipated from family, c̄ one sister who remains close and supportive, neighbor is a good friend and usually available to assist; both are currently out of town. Clara states, "It took a long time to get a ride here." To L&D c̄ friend.
   Smokes < 1 pack of cigarettes qd, 0 rx/recreational drugs, 0 ETOH, FOB [father of baby] unavailable.

Case Study 7.9a

1. Prioritize the objective and subjective data for written documentation.

OBJECTIVE	SUBJECTIVE
15 y/o	abd pain, cramping, vag pain
F	"my bladder hurts every time I pee"
75 kg	+ back pain
T 36°C po, P 105, R 20, BP 152/85	+ vaginal pain & cramping
FSBS 350	"My twin put me on insulin because
LNMP 12/98	the pills weren't working and she
DM II × 2 yrs	decides my sliding scale."
NKDA	

2. Write a verbal report for presentation to the nursing instructor.

   15 y/o F, admitted for candidal vaginitis & DM management, was left at the emergency room by mom with complaints of "bladder pain, abdominal pain, vaginal pain, and cramping," VS T 36°C, P 105, R 20, BP 152/85, LNMP 12/98, self-medicates with her mother's Vicodin 1 tab qd, past history includes DM II × 2 yrs., FSBS 350, takes glipizide 10 mg bid and insulin using a sliding scale determined by her twin, with no endocrine follow-up, asthma (RAD) inhaler Vanceril 2 puffs q6 hr and prn, no known drug allergies, P/SH: SW contacted mom who responds "Yeah, I know she is taking my insulin. I have DM and I know how much to give her," CPS referral

3. Write an admitting note.

   ID: 15 y/o, F, admit for candidal vaginitis & DM management
   CC: "bladder pain, abd pain, vag pain, & cramping"
   HPI: self medicates with her mother's Vicodin 1 tab qd
   VS: T 36°C, P 105, R 20, BP 152/85, LNMP 12/98
   PHx: DM II × 2 yrs., glipizide 10 mg bid, insulin based on sibling's sliding scale—endocrine f/u, FSBS 350

Asthma inhaler Vanceril 2 puffs q6 hr & prn, NKDA
Sliding scale: BS >95 5u reg
>200 15 u
>300 25 u
P/SH: CPS referral made, SW contacted mom who responded "Oh Lordy, not again" and "Yeah, I know she is taking my insulin. I have DM and I know how much to give her."

Case Study 7.9b

1. Write a discharge note for this patient.
   15 y/o F, admit via ER for candidal infection & DM II management 2 wks ago, DM controlled, FSBS 110, STD resolving. D'c to group home 15U NPH bid, glipizide 10 mg po bid, doxycycline 100 mg bid × 10 days, f/u c̄ endocrine clinic ×2 wks, f/u teen clinic STD & rape counseling. CPS to remain involved.

2. Write the following additional data for the CHH.
   General Appearance:
   15 y/o, 75 kg, age appropriate, quiet, friendly, cooperative, appears depressed, eyes directed to window, speaks only in response to question, no smiling
   Family History
   Mother: IDDM c R BKA
   Twin sister, 2 brothers DM II
   Personal/Social and Sexual History
   Lives c̄ mother, twin sister, and 2 brothers. Father peripherally involved. Teen's boyfriend is only support system. Hx significant for kidnap-assault-rape 10 mo past s̄ f/u counseling. She says "I still have flashbacks" and "Mom would never take me for counseling and she tells me all the time it was my fault and I deserved it." PH of suicidal attempt & ideation × 2 mos, attempt aborted by boyfriend. No subsequent attempts. Pt. well known to CPS r/t child abuse & neglect & med neglect referrals. (Mom responded to this referral, "Oh Lordy, not again.") Police hold @ pt request, secondary to hx. Teen states "I love my mom but I think I should have more help with this since I am only 15. I would rather go to a foster family."

Case Study 7.10a

1. Prioritize the objective and subjective data for written documentation.

OBJECTIVE	SUBJECTIVE
URI s/p 2 wks	"some swelling to the fingers"
Wt 13.8 kg	
BP 122/69, P 128, R 24, T 36.5°C ax	
NPO	
NKDA	
#3 Fr beveled perc line L AC (61 cm cath, 11 cm in, 50 cm out) flushed c̄ 100 u heparin/cc 3 cc s̄ resistance	
2 failed attempts R AC c̄ no BL	
oozing blood perc line insertion site	
EBL < 3 cc	

2. Write a verbal report for presentation to the nursing instructor.
   2 y/o M to room post I & D left calcaneus secondary to a 4-week history of osteomyelitis L heel, vital signs T 36.5°C ax, P 128, R 24, BP 122/69, wt. 13.8 kg, NPO, #3 French beveled percutaneous line left antecubital, flushed with 100 u heparin/cc 3 cc without resistance after 2 failed attempts R, estimated 3 cc blood noted perc line insertion site, pediatric nurse practitioner consulted, direct pressure for 15 min. to control blood loss, pressure dressing applied,

swelling observed fingers L hand. PHH pertinent for three ED visits times 4 weeks related to left calcaneus pain, upper respiratory infection times two weeks.

Case Study 7.10b

1. Write a follow-up narrative note.
   0900: afebrile, cultures pending, + CMS L ft, Kefzol infusing R AC perc line, PIV @ 40 gtt, Tyco elixir pain relief, ortho MD in at 0800.
   1000: PNP consulted, assessment R arm, notes swelling, tightness, & redness fingers to upper arm, gown removal revealed swelling from R shoulder/upper chest to below R nipple line. + dependent edema lateral & posterior to R shoulder blade, R AC perc line d'c'd, bevel tip intact c̄ line 61 cm tip to end, warm compress applied, to repeat q 1°, c̄ arm assessment, suspect poor line placement, parents supported & educated.

Case Study 7.10c

1. Write a follow-up narrative note.
   1200: Warm compress, T 100.3°F, ↓ irritability, ↑ po intake. + culture Staph C −

Case Study 7.10d

1. Write a follow-up narrative note.
   1. 1600: ↓ swelling, ↑ activity R arm, Tylenol c̄ relief, po's c̄ no difficulty, PIV patent & infusing, afebrile, warm compresses, child smiling & laughing.

Case Study 7.10e

1. Write a follow-up narrative note.
   1. 2200: L foot & R hand CMS no Δ, L PIV infusing s̄ problems, Kefzol, Tylenol pain, fluid reabsorbing c̄ ↓ swelling chest & shoulder, ↓ irritability, smiling at staff, parents appears more comfortable and relaxed.

CHAPTER 8

Medical and Legal Aspects of Documentation

WORD LIST

insult	force	abandonment
integrity	intervention	scope
illness	compensation	standard
injury	elopement	

 Exercise 8.1

Each item in the word list has both common and technical meanings. Match each word with its corresponding set of definitions and compare the intent or usage of the terms as both common and technical words.

1. _____

   Common: sickness
   Technical: abnormal process that interrupts or diminishes a person's functioning

2. _____

   Common: wound or damage; injustice
   Technical: any environmental interruption in a person's ability to adapt or defend state of well-being

3. _____

   Common: coming between or interference
   Technical: action to alter or modify a process

4. _____

   Common: run away to get married
   Technical: patient who leaves against medical recommendation or secretly

5. _____

   Common: strength or power; compel or inflict against resistance; large group
   Technical: to introduce food through tube to one unwilling or unable to eat

6. _____

   Common: honesty; strict values
   Technical: soundness of structure, unimpaired

7. _____

   Common: reimbursement
   Technical: counterbalance; adjustment for defect

8. _____

   Common: desert
   Technical: not fulfilling obligation toward patient

9. _____

   Common: the range of action or thought
   Technical: instrument for viewing or listening; a range that sets practice parameters

10. _____

    Common: flags or emblem; criterion
    Technical: minimum level used for basis of comparison

11. _____

    Common: derogatory reference to another or to self
    Technical: break in integrity; traumatic event

LEGAL ISSUES AND DOCUMENTATION

Nursing practice standards, hospital accreditation issues, and the potential for litigation make it necessary for nurses to review charting and evaluate if the written record complies with documentation standards. This chapter expands the concept of combining the consistent and technical use of language tools with a formatted style and developing a personal documentation model. This formatted model would emphasize the application of language to articulate patient care events or practices for notation in the medical record in keeping with regulatory, legal, and quality requirements.

The basis of any evaluation of patient care will involve a thorough review of the nurse's charting. Actual patient outcome and the documented record of care are the two primary indicators to determine if standards of practice were followed. The key between patient outcome and medical record is the application and influence of language. Good care is reflected with good charting. Good charting reflects good care practices. Good care practices, however, do not always ensure a good patient outcome. Language used in the medical record establishes that standards were observed and is used by a judge or jury to evaluate the standard of care even if the patient outcome was not positive.

It is fair to state that the potential for legal consequences based upon the content of a nurse's documentation must be given consideration. It is a good habit for nurses to chart as if they were planning on reading the note three or more years later. Ask yourself if what you are documenting today would present a clear, relevant, and complete account several years from now if the record were

---

BOX 8.1

Expert Witness Testimony

Nurses may be subpoenaed to deliver expert witness testimony in a court of law. The potential for being deposed and being a witness may be in criminal or civil court, or possibly in license review by a professional board. Many nurses are called on to testify before legislative committees that are investigating medical issues. They may testify at arbitration hearings regarding labor disputes.

The testifying nurse often relies on the language and completeness of documentation, either his or her own or that which is under review. Most nurses work their whole career without involvement in court or legislative testimony. It is prudent to learn to write clear notes in the event that this may occur. Relying on memory of a specific incident or patient is inappropriate and dangerous.

reviewed. But even more important perhaps is the concept that a nurse's note, written about a patient's course of medical care, regardless of the setting, will affect the nature and appropriateness of the care given. Documentation needs to be accurate, complete, and objective as well as defensible regardless of who is reading and interpreting the note.

In the preceding chapters emphasis has been placed on the importance of a complete note. This includes all aspects necessary to understand the course of an event or patient care. To summarize the assessment, planning, implementation, outcome, and evaluation of the outcome are non-negotiable components of any personal documentation model. Each charting entry must be a complete entity and must reflect both medically and legally the course of patient events.

A nurse's subjective and objective observations are valid. Remember that the presentation of such information must be made with measurable descriptors. Words must be selected to remove any bias or emotionality from the record of care. In chapters 4 and 5 you learned about the specific and descriptive use of language and objective data and to employ appropriate, clear parameters to use with the more subjective data in order to recreate the picture of the patient situation upon which the care is based. The word picture you recreate must be without bias, and subjective statements must be supported with objective assessment data. Consistency in the presentation of data adds to the credibility of the recorder and implies a pattern of clear and organized thinking. A standardized, professional approach toward managing patient care regardless of the chaos that may characterize critical medical situations helps to establish a standardized, recorded model that will hold up to medical or legal review even years after the patient visit.

The charting samples at the end of this chapter are examples of clear, defensible documentation.

Nurses must review their attitudes and approach with regard to patient documentation. Why do nurses need to chart? To what end does the patient record serve? As we reflect on practical and legal mandates, charting changes from a nuisance "chore" to a viable "tool" with which to describe events or care. Documentation becomes a more dynamic model using language "techniques" to communi-

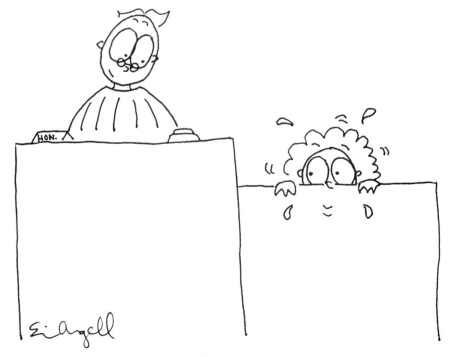

The Judge

cate among other members of the health care team. Through practice, nurses will standardize the format in which they chart to conform with the accreditation and regulatory requirements of their facility. Such standardized practice will promote efficiency in the written record and satisfy quality and continuity of care needs.

DEFENSIBLE CONTENT

The content of a nurse's notes must be written with an eye toward patient outcome, both in the "best case" or "worst case" scenario. The same content should also be defensible when reviewed by a colleague or a legal consultant who is dissecting a chart for litigation purposes. This includes both the content of the charted note and the data which is absent. The adage "If it wasn't charted, it wasn't done" is almost impossible to avoid if legal review is undertaken. It may seem far-fetched to be accountable for what was not noted in your documentation, but it is not. Attorneys will recreate a "picture" for a jury based on what is included in the record. Patient events, either confirmed or not denied in the patient's medical record, will be used to recount an occurrence.

Noting the sequence of events as related to the care of a patient is in keeping with standards for nursing practice for an individual patient scenario and is a critical component of the quality evaluation process. An accurate and complete sequence of events will also be critical in defending choices and care should the case come for legal review.

BOX 8.2

Language Pitfalls and the Law

Words are necessary to concise and clear charting. But when do words present a potential legal problem? By now, it should be clear that word omission, unsubstantiated subjectivity, and misspellings can potentially obstruct appropriate care and lead to legal misinterpretation. Misuse of terms and vague description applied to signs and symptoms may create deviations from an ideal care plan. Biased characterization of a patient, or the patient's compliance to recommended care, is generally problematic and does not have a place in the medical record.

Individual words may also be misused, even by the expert nurse. Some words can be used as descriptor or as diagnosis. For instance, the word *anxiety* is frequently used in describing a patient's affect, often without substantiating objective data. The ordinary nurse using this term may be viewed as diagnosing without license to do so. A psychiatric nurse practitioner, on the other hand, may be well qualified to diagnose the patient if the criteria that validates the diagnosis are present and documented. The problem of diagnosis may be solved if a patient meets the criteria for the nursing diagnosis, "anxiety, related to."

The following words may be problematic depending on the context in which they are used, or the objective data necessary to support their use:

dehydration

diarrhea

inflammation

ecchymosis

apnea

Nurses can use fluid volume deficit, actual or potential for, as a reasonable substitute for dehydration, which might be regarded as a diagnosis. Be aware that this is a term that may be frequently used by nurse. No problems may result from the use until a lawsuit is filed. If a nurse has used the word *dehydration* and all potential interventions are not documented in resolving the problem, the nurse could be stuck in a legal quagmire. For example, a reasonable intervention for dehydration would be infusion of hydrating solution. If, in fact, the record shows isotonic solution was administered instead, the intervention may be viewed as not within an acceptable standard. The solution is to choose words carefully. Document objective data in appropriate detail. Be clear and specific.

The Board of Registered Nursing identifies practice standards and expectations. JCAHO outlines documentation standards that must be met for facility accreditation. Medicare requires certain elements of documentation be met in order to obtain reimbursement. The basis for effective documentation be it for legal, financial, or quality purposes is, in fact, the use of language.

The use of language, its absence, that which is inappropriate or could be misinterpreted, spelling (that emphasizes the attention to detail) and the legibility of the record all affect the nurse's ability to defend the content of the chart. Often, the impact of the defense of a record's content can be correlated to the impact on a patient's care, positive or negative.

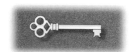

Which words, used in what manner, are the keys to defensible charting? There are as many and varied answers as there are patients. However, the medical record of care must accurately and succinctly reflect patient care practices. The language a nurse uses to chart must demonstrate that prudent, medically necessary, and reasonable care standards were observed and applied as indicated by the patient's status or condition. A complete and accurate medical record of events will likely satisfy insurance reimbursement needs. The use of objective, consistent, and professional language is a key concept to charting in a manner that will also describe the care events should a quality or legal review occur.

INDIVIDUAL RESPONSIBILITY

Nurses are responsible for the content of their own charting. In any litigation, a nurse is bound by their Nursing Practice Act. Just as the Board of Nursing has the responsibility to interpret and enforce the standards of the Act, an individual nurse has the responsibility to observe and practice within the standards of the Act. In general, a nurse has the duty to deliver ordinary or reasonable care that a reasonable and prudent nurse would employ under similar circumstances.

BOX 8.3

Who Is a "Reasonable and Prudent" Nurse?

There are many levels of nursing education. Nursing education is disparate, and graduate nurses hold many different degrees. Diploma, or hospital-based, nursing programs are almost completely phased out in the United States. Nurses in most states are qualified to sit for board exams after completing associate degree (ADN), bachelor's degree (BSN), or master's (MSN) nursing programs. There are also nurses from other countries and from the military who may take the boards. Advanced practice nurses and clinical specialists add another layer to the level of expertise among staff. Specialty certification is also available to nurses from the American Nurses Association or from a specialty's governing organization, for example, flight nurses.

All nurses are expected to be held to the "usual or ordinary" nurse standard relating to the area of care the nurse is presently working in and the policies governing nursing practices. If any nurse, with minimal experience, can reasonably be expected to know how to respond to a given circumstance, the "usual" nurse standard applies. The ordinary nurse is also expected to conform to laws of practice and patient advocacy. A nurse must exercise prudent and informed judgment when initiating care or making decisions on behalf of his or her patients. A nurse will be held accountable to his or her level of training and to the Nurse Practice Act. A nurse is also responsible to know and observe the policies and procedures of the work unit. A nurse with advanced licensure or specialty certification will be held to standards that are higher than those expected of the usual and ordinary nurse.

All nurses are expected to document in a professional manner. **It is considered usual and prudent nursing practice to include appropriate information in a clear and concise manner.**

If a nurse practices outside of the scope of the Nursing Practice Act or outside the scope of his or her employment, an act of malpractice may have been incurred by that nurse.

Employers may or may not choose to defend a nurse who is involved in a patient incident that resulted in litigation. If an act of malpractice has been committed, the employer is not likely to support the nurse in the event of error outside of the Nurse Practice Act. The nurse's primary tool in defending any expected or unexpected event is through the written, recorded course of events.

Most nurses understand that omissions in charting, subjective or vague language, improper error notations, illegal abbreviations, spelling and grammatical errors, and illegible writing do not support the "reasonable and prudent" standard of practice dictums. At the same time, these are among the most commonly accepted errors permitted in charting by nurses. Even if a care setting does not provide the nurse with an adequate system for recording data, or proper documentation tools in which to record accurate data and prioritize the importance of solid documentation, the nurse still has an individual responsibility to ensure that documentation, like nursing care, conforms to the "reasonable and prudent" standard.

COST RECOVERY AND DOCUMENTATION

A nurse's documentation can adversely affect the ability of the institution to recover costs of care from private and public insurance payers. This impact may also be felt by the patient, who may bear the cost of denied charges. Our professional documentation needs to minimize the financial impact to both health care delivery system and recipient. A nurse's most trusted responsibility is the welfare of his or her patient. In this regard, the nurse takes on the role of the patient's advocate. As such, nurses are required to act in the best interests of their patients.

To deliver good care is no longer good enough. Today's nurse must also document such care, be cost effective in delivering that patient care, and intervene for the patient to limit and avoid negative outcomes.

Once again, the key influence in the recording of such care is the use of language to describe and record into the chart a sequence of patient events. Legibility, attention to grammar and spelling, and the proper use of descriptive terms are critical factors in legal and sound charting. It is the individual nurse's professionally licensed responsibility to make every charting entry a valid one.

ERROR, ERROR!

As long as there are human caregivers there will be the risk for error in caregiving or in documenting the care that was given. There are proper ways to initially record data and there are appropriate methods to correct errors in both delivery of care and data documentation. The physician must be notified in the event of an error in the delivery of care, and that notification must be documented. The manner in which to record or note an incident or error is very specific in form and content. Any nurse will commit errors during the course of his or her professional career. It is as important to observe standards for care and charting as it is to observe requirements to correct errors in documentation.

The use of incident reports, quality management notification forms, or assignment despite objection forms are a part of daily operations in any busy health care setting. The language a nurse uses must reflect as objectively as possible the actual sequence of events as noted by that observer. As a part of any nurse's personal documentation model, it is critical to know how to record incidents, correct

BOX 8.4

Assignment Despite Objection

Given increasing patient acuity in conjunction with critical care nursing shortages, nurses may feel required by employers to assume excessive patient assignments or to care for patients whose acuity exceeds the nurse's area of expertise or experience. Individual settings may not offer appropriate avenues for the nurse to document how the assignment might be inappropriate or the nurse's reluctance to accept the assignment. Once a nurse has reported to work, refusing a patient or assignment might be interpreted as abandonment. Accepting an assignment that the nurse is not qualified to care for might result in malpractice. What to do?

If you need to complete a risk or quality notification form where you work, it is a good idea to keep copies of any inappropriate assignment reports or other practice issues that you submit to the employer. In a court of law, the recognition of unsafe conditions must be accompanied by proof that the nurse has made a reasonable attempt to correct the situation. Keeping accurate records of these events may even demonstrate that the employer's usual practice showed a pattern of abuse. Be aware of the "whistleblower" protection in each state in which you practice. If an employer demonstrates a pattern of poor practice, your continued employment, while you express concern about the care provided, may raise questions about your own standards.

There are reasons that nurses remain working for these employers: long-term employment, retirement vesting, change in quality of care during long-term employment, desire to protect patients within the system, and desire to effect system change from within. It is vital that nurses who continue to work in questionable institutions know the risks and are prepared to explain their rationale. The risk of litigation increases if poor practice by nursing or medical staff is overlooked or accepted by the facility.

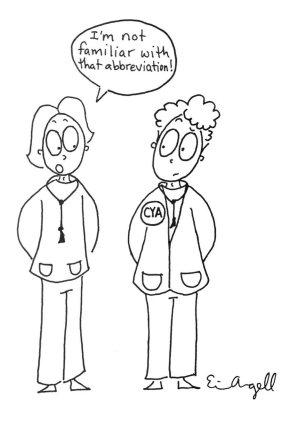

errors, or make changes or additions to the medical record. Just as a nurse will develop a formatted style in which to accomplish routine documentation entries, a nurse can also learn effective strategies in which to record unexpected events or errors. Later in this chapter, discussion will focus on such processes as a part of the nurse's language application model for documentation of patient care practices.

GOOD DATA, RECORDED WISELY

Effective use of language is the best way to ensure that the data you have gathered in the clinical setting are used to enhance patient care and to protect the nurse or health care facility from legal jeopardy.

The basic principles observed by nurses when documenting in a patient's medical record remain constant between texts and experts who teach nurses how to chart. Key among these standards for charting are consistency and completeness.

In other words, in the event of any patient outcome, good or bad, expected or unexpected, a nurse will be held accountable for care rendered or care withheld. Judges and juries will refer to the medical record to determine that patient's status before, during, and after an event and in determining if an error of commission or act of omission transpired. The nurse who has used a standardized and professional format to document circumstances, which thoroughly and concisely depicts events, will be able to reflect patient care standards he or she used. It is in the review of the documented record that standards of care are either evident or lacking.

Throughout this text, you have been learning to discriminate, using language to selectively choose words to associate your documentation with a standard of care. Nowhere is it more important to observe such differentiation in language as it is during a legal review of care given to any patient. If nurses suspected in advance of the care rendered that the medical record would be reviewed, would the charting be different? The answer is often "yes" but should in fact and practice be "no." Any documentation by any nurse should be able to withstand a legal review at any time. Sadly, many nurses simply do not anticipate or appreciate the potential for medical or legal review at the time of their documentation efforts, and charting submitted to the record more often reflects the absence of good documentation habits.

Why then does more than one standard exist? One possibility is the difficulty of the job today's nurses must perform. The workplace environment in the contemporary health care market is extremely challenging and does not support efficiency at many levels. Another possibility is that nurses are simply not adequately prepared to know, with certainty, what constitutes complete, accurate charting. Charting is a skill that many nurses "pick up" as they proceed through school or in their first years at employment. Many good and bad habits are learned by nurses. Compounded by a difficult work environment and the mandate for written notes, one understands why the charting process itself is ripe for error.

Earlier in this chapter, the importance of a personal documentation model was acknowledged. At this point, let's discuss how language must be applied to support a nurse's personal documentation model and must also reflect that individual nurse's patient care choices and practices.

CHARTING STYLE

How do nurses learn good charting? When do nurses learn good charting? Where do nurses learn about good charting? Every nurse has a personal documentation style, a format for charting all of their own. Even if the facility the nurse works for uses a standardized charting method such as "narrative" or "SOAP," no one is standing over the nurse as pen is put to paper or fingers to computer keyboard. No one assists the nurse in selecting which words to relate the sequence of a patient event.

There are "teachable moments" at every turn, but often no time or teacher present to teach. While in clinical rotations during school, student nurses learn by their instructor's intervention or by observing examples of charting in the patient's record. Part of the problem associated with this learning style is that the observed example in the medical record may be a poor one or the instructor is unable to make time to emphasize and correlate the patient care intervention with proper supportive documentation.

New nurses who are in their first few years of employment go on further to add to their style of personal documentation by following example, by taking continuing education classes, or by simply repeating habits already learned. The important point to recognize is that nurses possess a personal format and style for documentation. Whether good or bad, complete or incomplete, supportive or nonsupportive, nurses do make entries into the medical record every shift. As such, it is incumbent upon individual nurses to learn techniques that will document, demonstrate, and support the care given in the event of inquiry or review.

LANGUAGE APPLICATION MODEL FOR NURSE PRACTICE

There are four elements of the language application documentation model. These four factors interrelate to support complete and accurate documentation. Whatever the patient outcome, only the written documentation will support that the standard of care was rendered.

One of the four elements of the language application model relates directly to patient care. This element is labeled "quality of care requirements" and has to do with those aspects, both expected and unexpected, of the patient's care which transpired during the patient's stay. The other three factors of the documentation model are standards for language use in charting; requirements for reimbursement strategies; and legal standards for chart review.

Figure 8.1
Language Model for Patient Care Practice

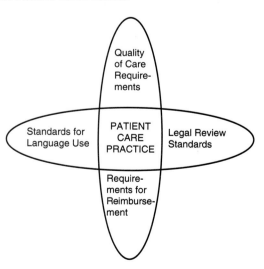

As nurses learn to differentiate within the technical language of medicine and apply words discriminatingly to the patient's written record, that nurse adds to his or her experiential base for documentation standards. Discussion in this chapter is intended to add to a nurse's knowledge base regarding the differentiation and a more selective language application process as related to the four elements of the personal documentation model. Let's first begin with quality of care requirements.

QUALITY OF CARE REQUIREMENTS

As previously mentioned the Nurse Practice Act, JCAHO, and the state's Board of Registered Nursing are among the entities that define standards of practice for nurses and health care facilities. All nurses are accountable to that standard whether they are aware of the standard or not.

In the aspect of the personal documentation model, the quality of care requirements have been defined by the regulating bodies mentioned earlier, and a nurse is responsible to observe charting practices that support the defined patient care standard.

As such, the nurse is responsible to both maintain and document the expected standard for care. Related to the language application documentation model, how does a nurse chart what is necessary and expected to demonstrate that safe patient care was administered? The answer rests within the standards of practice.

BOX 8.5

E-Documentation and "Shadow" Charts

Nurses are becoming familiar with electronic charting. Some hospitals and clinics have been using only computers for many years. Handheld computers are being used at the bedside.

There are many advantages in using bedside e-documentation. Data are entered immediately, charges may be automatic. Electronic forms, however, may not be equipped with a section for necessary narrative. Computers cannot know what is intended if a word is misspelled or entered in error. Systems should time-date and add corrections to the chart, but the computer cannot know for certain who is entering the information. If there is a central data bank, a computer problem can limit access to necessary information.

Some providers are keeping "shadow" charts to feel secure about having patient information available in the event of data retrieval problem. Nurses may be compelled to keep journals or patient notes if they feel that data are incomplete or that the system chosen by the facility is unreliable.

There will be many issues with e-documentation that will be overlooked until an event occurs that brings the problem to the attention of health care providers.

Nursing education programs must start by incorporating the standards for patient care into their teaching curricula. The care being taught should be based in the defined practice standards. The unifying "language" between instructors teaching and students learning is in fact language itself. Throughout this book you have been learning that words must be selected carefully, with consideration toward their specific and technical application to the patient's chart. Chapters 4 and 5 introduced the key concept that you must use words and descriptors to most appropriately describe and record actions. Your findings must avoid personal bias or the use of trigger words, which might be interpreted by another health care provider to adversely affect the patient's care.

The first element of the documentation model defines itself in its name, "quality of care requirements." It is about knowing standard for care as well as being able to discriminate between our common and technical language to use words that describe the standard of care given to the patient.

Some of the habits you can use to better define and develop your personal documentation have been previously mentioned. The use of descriptors or modifiers when charting and familiarity with your facility's policies and procedures are two key habits to incorporate in daily practice. Chapter 5 reminded you that a primary responsibility of any nurse is that of patient advocate. The Nurse Practice Acts direct nurses to act as the client's advocate and initiate actions to either improve care or to avoid care that is against the patient's better interests. Our professional nursing license obligates us to observe the "Patient Bill of Rights" on behalf of our patients. As patient care progresses or patient events and outcomes occur, entries into the medical record, the only recorded account, provide dimension and detail to the quality of care rendered.

BOX 8.6

Advocacy

Nurses have a primary role as patient advocates. This role may be written into the state Nursing Practice Act. Section 1443.5, Part 6 of the Nursing Practice Act of California, which lists the standards of competent performance, reads:

(6) Acts as the client's advocate, as circumstances require, by initiating action to improve health care or to change decisions or activities which are against the interests of the client, and by giving the client the opportunity to make informed decisions about health care before it is provided.

It does not say that the nurse makes judgments or decisions for the patient. It does not say that the nurse approves of the patient or defends a patient's behavior. It doesn't even say that the nurse needs to assume responsibility beyond his or her own scope of practice, such as being the agent of rather than the witness for "informed consent."

Nurses who question the appropriateness of medical care yet fail to write a quality assurance report, who neglect to record errors on an incident report, or who accept assignments inconsistent with their scope of practice without documented objection, may not be meeting this standard of competence.

Each state's Nursing Practice Act is different. It is imperative that nurses learn how the scope of practice is defined for their state. Most Nursing Practice Acts are written in legal language. Language, as always, is the key to understanding the act. If necessary attend workshops in order to protect your practice.

As a nurse, you have a professional responsibility to address, with your patients, issues of informed consent, refusal of treatment, advanced directives, refusal of medical screening exam, and leaving the hospital against medical advice. Each of these issues is under the area of quality of care and carries a strong potential for review of practice, especially in the event of a bad outcome during a procedure. In order to ensure that your legal responsibilities were met on behalf of your patient, there are a few basic considerations for assuring completeness and accuracy of the previously mentioned forms.

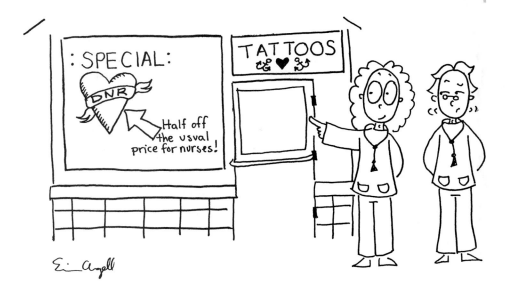

First, the patient's signature represents the patient's acknowledgment that he or she understands the language on the form or paper they are signing. Be sure that you use common language to explain to the patient what he or she is signing. Do not change what is on the form. If you are changing words to provide verbal explanation for the patient's understanding, always note the exact words of your explanation on the back of the form or consent.

For example, if a patient does not comprehend the term "lumbar puncture," you can "interpret" the procedure for the patient. You might instead say, "The doctor uses a small needle to poke a tiny hole into the skin near your tailbone. The doctor calls that a lumbar puncture and that is what he thinks he needs to do in order to find out what is wrong with your baby." Such interpretation recreates a visual image for the patient's better understanding. Remember, it is critical to associate your interpretation with the words on the consent or refusal form. If the patient were asked to restate what they were told, any interpretation you provide for the patient must in fact represent the nature of the consent or

---

BOX 8.7

Informed Consent

Just for fun, take a moment to consider how you might describe the following patient care procedures or treatments in order to promote informed consent. Discuss with your peers what words may best describe the procedures. In many cases, the physician may have already explained the procedure to the patient. If, however, the illness or injury is an emergency or the patient has questions, nurses may be involved with obtaining the patient's consent. Remember, it is important to avoid bias words when providing an explanation, to refer serious questions or patient concerns to the physician, and always try to provide the patient with ample opportunity to make his or her decision.

Intravenous administration of chemotherapeutic agents

Intravenous pyelorogram

Computerized tomography of abdomen

Tetanus vaccination

Open reduction and internal fixation

Transurethral prostatectomy

Chest tube insertion

Liver BIOPSY

Circumcision

Total abdominal hysterectomy

Suture repair of facial laceration

procedure. This example indeed reflects more of a layperson's description of a lumbar puncture procedure and would likely help the patient understand the physician's recommendation.

A second important habit to develop for the quality of care element of the documentation model is based in nursing practice. Whether you work in an acute or subacute area, it is your personal responsibility to understand the professional requirements of your practice and license. Whether your nursing assessment is connected with a nursing diagnosis, patient care plan, or clinical pathway, at some point your care must be connected to a plan of care that also provides for implementation and evaluation of that care.

Nurse's notes reflect your assessment, planning, and evaluation process. They "tell" the story of your plan of care. Be familiar with and understand the policies and procedures for the facility in which you are working. If you happen to work in a specialty area outside of the usual scope of nursing practice, as in obstetrics or sexual assault, then you must know with certainty the policies for your specialty area of practice. How can a nurse begin to know what to document if he or she does not know the policies under which they work? All nurses enter practice with an ability to use language. The key concept with quality of care is, in fact, quality. You must know the quality aspects of your job before you can successfully apply language in a quality manner.

BOX 8.8

Journals

There is some controversy over the wisdom of nurses keeping personal journals to record incidents they believe may be reviewed by either hospital committees or for litigation. There are two alternate views:

1. There is never too much documentation. Memory is unreliable at best and perceptions of an incident change as staff members review and discuss the event.
2. It is best to rely only on the legal written record. If facts are forgotten or if uncertainty about the sequence of events exists, it is best to rely on saying that you do not recall a specific item.

There is also the question of keeping separate records, which may be subpoenaed. All of your journals may become public record. Journal keeping is a very personal decision made by individual nurses with or without the aid of counsel.

A third important aspect for the quality element of the documentation model is in selecting words to describe nursing assessment data. As licensed nurses, we are educated and qualified to conduct a nursing assessment. We record statements from the patient about the history of the present illness (HPI), relating that illness with a review of the patient's systems (ROS), and then perform an assessment of the patient's physical systems. As part of the complete health history (CHH), we measure the patient's vital signs, listen to lungs, assess aspects of growth and development, relate aspects of growth and development to age-related behaviors, and assess the patient's status of circulation and mentation.

These assessments are performed in order to make a nursing-based diagnosis (NANDA) and to implement a plan for nursing care. They are not done in order to "figure out what the patient has"; that is for the physician to determine. A nurse must enter his or her nursing assessment as a permanent part of the patient's medical record.

When selecting words to describe nursing assessment data, remember that nurses do not diagnose. Consider the potential of the subjectively based entry, "fussy baby," versus the more objectively recorded "Child being held by mother. Unable to distract, crying tears, and mother unable to console." In the first notation (depending upon the child's age) the physician may be obligated to perform a medical workup to rule out meningitis. There is nothing in the charting to support a physical or emotional basis for the child's distress.

BOX 8.9

Differentiation, Not Diagnosis

The following are samples of common charting entries in many patient records. As you read them, consider your own practice and habits. Are there areas of your documentation in which subjective statements are submitted as "fact"? It is quite possible, as it is difficult to quantify many aspects of the patient's assessment or complaint. Remember the liability and additional, unnecessary expense such subjective entries impose on the physician and health care system. To improve your personal habits, first isolate and identify such subjective entries in your charting and consider what it is you are trying to communicate. Work to quantify those areas where you can correlate subjective statements with measurement scales and place patient statements in quotation marks where you cannot correlate data.

Chest pain

Slept through the night

Tolerated procedure well

Looked pale

Appears very short of breath

No complaints

Complains of slight abdominal pain

Small amount bright red bloody drainage noted postpartum

Refused injection

Sleepy in recovery room

Compare the two examples. The second example associates observations as to patient behavior "unable to distract or console" with related physical findings "being held by mother, crying tears." The first entry could be interpreted in at least four ways, including a child with meningitis, a nurse being impatient with a scared child, a child with a fever and not feeling physically well, or a child who does not especially enjoy visits to the doctor. It is also a prime example of nurses turning assessments into medical diagnoses.

To make the first statement immediately more clear and less subjective or biased, the nurse could add the following: mother states, "fussy baby." Take a moment to consider the adverse potential of such statements. Nurses are qualified to record related events, nurses are not qualified to make medical diagnoses. When necessary or indicated, use the patient's exact words in quotation marks to describe or support your nursing assessment. This will almost always help you to avoid inaccurate or biased interpretations of your documentation. This is a key point in this first element of the personal documentation model.

> ### BOX 8.10
> ## Drawing Conclusions
>
> Another problem area is documenting in a manner that assumes a conclusion. If you chart that a patient is "not responding" to an intervention, you have inadvertently drawn a conclusion. It is far more appropriate to document that expected outcomes from a procedure or medication are absent. For instance, if you administer a medication to reduce a fever and the patient's temperature remains the same or increases, the data themselves objectify the lack of response to the fever medication.
>
> Other conclusions might include psychosocial issues, societal judgment, and racial bias. These conclusions may be used to imply that the nurse has demonstrated that he or she offers disparate treatment to patients based on personal interpretation or bias.

STANDARDS FOR LANGUAGE IN DOCUMENTATION

The second element of the model involves the standard for language used in documentation. It also involves reviewing how words are actually put on paper. Your charting must provide an appropriate description of what transpired, of what the patient needed, if events occurred outside of routine or expected occurrence, and in a timely and chronological manner. This second aspect of the personal documentation model includes the tenets that are standard to good documentation. Along with a selective discrimination process among common and technical language, this element addresses what is important about how you use words to document a sequence of patient events.

All of the teaching points you might learn in a course about documentation are relevant. One of the more important rules for good charting is to chart everything, your observations and actions. Note the patient's symptoms or complaints and use the patient's own words. Document what you did for the patient and how the patient responded every time and any time you gave medications or treatments. Mention any safety precautions you took and efforts you made to contact physicians. Make your signature and title complete and legible.

The key to these rules for charting, which best serves this second element, standard of language, is the application of language to describe events. Correct spelling, proper use of grammar and punctuation, use of facility-approved abbreviations, and being familiar with the policies the facility uses are all vital to the successful execution of this element.

Most nurses know practitioners who have illegible handwriting or who are poor spellers. We shake our heads, get impatient, and ask for clarification over and over again. Think of examples that demonstrate these bad habits and then imagine them enlarged for an overhead presentation in a courtroom. It is no wonder that large monetary awards are frequently granted in malpractice lawsuits.

It seems obvious to state that a complete and sequential recording of events, legibility, and correct spelling are necessary to a professional presentation of your documentation. It is also true that nurses work in a stressful and challenging work environment. Corners are cut and "less than perfect" is, at times, accepted. So it goes with our own personal documentation. If a nurse has to endure the experience of a legal deposition or a courtroom appearance, he or she will find a way to avoid cutting corners and alter poor personal practice habits permanently.

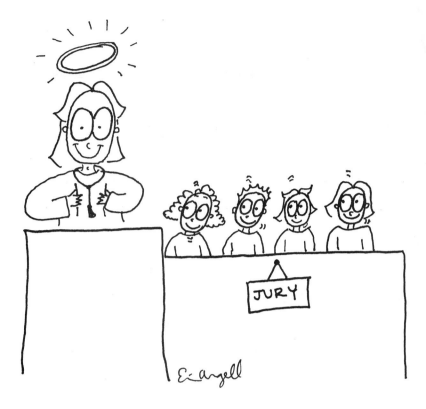

BOX 8.11

Forensic Charting

Forensics is the relationship between medical data and legal process. Nurses working in the ER, OR, occupational health, and as suspected assault examiners must be aware of the legal implications of their written notes. Nurses who work with such patient cases must be aware that the content of their notes affects the outcome of potential future criminal investigations.

It is not unusual for the layperson to link the term *forensic* only with criminal investigations or with investigations of the medical examiner. Nurses, however, must be aware that there are frequent occasions in which their documentation is forensic in nature and may be involved in a future legal case. The obvious example is the medical care for victims and perpetrators of crimes. From the emergency department visit to discharge from extended rehabilitation, all data may be included in the ultimate resolution of a criminal case. Documentation of the appearance of injury, procedure necessary to treat an injury, as well as how the injury may have affected the procedure are part of the necessary data. Likewise, all data gathered following motor vehicle accidents, possible domestic violence, and suspected child neglect and abuse are relevant to the legal investigation.

Operating room personnel often care for victims and perpetrators of violence. Documentation of the appearance of injury and the procedure, as well as how the injury may have affected the procedure, are part of the necessary data.

Occupational illness and injury involves keeping accurate records to determine the cause of a work-related illness or injury as well as for prevention of like incidents. Worker safety is a public health problem prior to occurrence, a legal problem after occurrence, and an ongoing problem for an injured worker.

Is there something in between bad practice and a courtroom drama? How do we motivate ourselves to do what is necessary and not cut critical corners? Start with what you are documenting and review your own standard for legibility and spelling. By being aware and reviewing what you are currently doing, there is tremendous opportunity to improve with no extra effort. Just ensure the legibility and spelling of what you are currently noting. It may take extra work at first to find the common and medical dictionaries on your unit and to learn to incorporate their use into your time management practices. It's easier to ask someone how to spell words and is occasionally the practical solution. But for frequent or chronic misspellers, learning to use a dictionary may be your only recourse to working well with your peers.

Every nurse makes notes in the medical record. Whether acknowledged or not, every nurse has a personal documentation model. By taking a moment to review what you currently enter into the medical record, you can begin to focus attention on your personal format. To correct spelling and legibility errors is a very important first step in learning how to better improve your overall charting and documentation habits.

A second point to emphasize in learning how to better select and apply words in your personal model for documentation is to begin with what is obvious. Your first efforts to turn attention to the details of spelling and legibility will also help you to focus on what you are saying in the record. What you are saying about the patient may then focus your attention on what you are not saying about the patient. Just as patient care events occur in a sequential manner, documentation also happens in an ordered, structured, and sequential format.

This strategy for learning about the element standard for language use is based in description and sequential order. Be certain about the timing and occurrence of patient events. Know what is important to record and match it with a descriptive word you've selected to document the sequence of events. Selectively choose words, and before you ever make a charting entry, consider what it is you want to

---

BOX 8.12

Words Badly Spelled

The following examples were collected by the authors from charting samples. They represent some of the more humorous ways in which words are misspelled. As far-fetched as these samples may seem, they are taken from actual patient records. Remember also that nurses have a mandate to practice like their peers and in accordance to reasonable standards. Consider the opportunity to discredit the nurse, in comparison with his or her peers, in front of a jury if such poor spelling is permitted into the patient's legal record of care.

emmissis

cronic

ambilatory

alzhermeirz

justational diabitic

boad & care home

trama

darreha

fuzzy baby

preasure

baged for urin

dauter

duaghter

aperant

apeared

en-root

en-rout

grimises

oder

flemm

flemn

hystaria

say. What must you include, what do you not need to include? What is relevant to the patient's care and outcome? What nursing actions do you need to relate? What patient picture do you want to recreate? Just because nurses notes are silent doesn't mean there isn't anything to say.

Accreditation surveyors, quality managers, and juries all rely on the patient's medical record to tell them what went on at the patient's bedside. Begin learning about your own mode of documentation by first reviewing your personal habits of spelling and legibility. Then, continue learning by considering what it is you actually need to communicate, to "say," to any future reviewer of the patient's record. The exercises in Chapter 4 regarding the use of descriptors and avoiding bias will help you to better note what it is you want to say. The review of subjective versus objective word choices in Chapter 5 will also help you to make more prudent entries into the medical record.

The second element focuses on how words are put into the medical record. Words must be focused. Words must be specific. By using language objectively applied and specific to the event, nurses avoid vagueness and inconsistency in the record. It is important to recreate a clear, precise picture. It is important to avoid bias and trigger words. It is important to relate what the patient states in the patient's own words. It is important to do so in a timely and legible manner.

BOX 8.13

Can You Picture This?

When learning to use words to recreate a picture, consider what you want to say. Read your nurses notes to see if you have accomplished your goal. By reading your charting, even aloud if possible, you have an opportunity to review what you wanted or needed to say. Do your words meet or match your intent? Remember the "rules" about quantifying subjective statements and the use of quotation marks. To further paint your word picture, review your current charting practices.

The following samples are again taken from actual patient records. The potential for amusement does not protect against the potential for liability when being compared in a courtroom with a "reasonable standard" and "prudent peer" practice. One wonders if the authors of these samples would have better described the events and changed the word selection if they had taken just a moment to reread their entries.

"26 year old male reclining on left elbow and ground. Diagnosis: multiple gunshot wound to head and abdomen"

"36 year old male, some abdominal pain on palpation, no other complaint. Drank 1 quart tequila, friends carried inside to bed. Vomitus has odor of tequila"

"2 victims of motor vehicle accident, minor passenger space intrusion, no starred windshield. Major fracture to telephone pole"

"the lab test indicated abnormal lover function"

"the skin is moist and dry"

"she stated she had been constipated for most of her life"

"the patient suffers from occasional, constant, infrequent headaches"

"patient was alert and unresponsive"

LEGAL STANDARDS OF REVIEW

The third element of the personal documentation model involves the legal aspects of health care and charting. It is identified as the legal standards of review. The focus of this element is on charting practices that are specifically organized to support and record standard of care. How is nursing documentation related to patient events, care, and case reviews? Documentation in the medical record is acknowledged to be the primary means with which to review and evaluate patient occurrences. The patient's chart is a legal record of the patient's care. As such, the aspects of a nurse's charting become central and relevant should a chart be pulled for legal review.

The quality and language aspects of the personal documentation model have been reviewed. Chapter 3 discussed medical and legal considerations that indicate a need for a formatted style of documentation. Key to this third element is the necessity for personal documentation habits that follow a consistent format and employ basic documentation knowledge. However, just because a nurse charts well does not mean good care was given. And, because a nurse gives good care does not mean he or she charts well. Good documentation and good care are not mutually exclusive of each other but do, in fact, benefit from the same habits of a standardized approach.

The nurse with a systematic method, a "format" for patient assessment and planning care as well as for documentation, lays the foundation for excellence in practice. Documentation is the unifying factor between practice and patient care. Language use is the key in documentation. Nurses need and use systems to provide care. Personal documentation models also need a systematic approach. Complete, objective, and standardized charting represents a nurse's performance and attention to the quality and legal aspects of our patient care responsibilities.

The medical record is no place for inadequate or inaccurate documentation. Many lawsuits involve aspects of malpractice or negligence. Negligence is more often considered to be either acts of commission or errors of omission. That is, acts the nurse did, or failed to do, which fell below the standard of care as defined by the Nurse Practice Act.

Malpractice is more inclusive and involves improper or unprofessional conduct. There are many experts in the areas of negligence and malpractice, and our emphasis is on stressing awareness about these two legal problems.

Focus on the potential for legal consequences associated with a legal review of your personal method of charting. Look at the words you select to document data, the sequence, and the degree of completeness of your charting. You are learning to modify patient assessment data for definition and clarification based upon medical and legal considerations. The third element places the emphasis on learning a consistent method with which to document patient care. Develop a standardized format to use with your routine or exceptional charting.

Earlier you reviewed your current standard for spelling and grammar. You considered the impact of subjective charting entries. You even practiced rereading your entries to better understand what you would like to state in the record. Next, incorporate a standardized order, a format, in how you make actual entries in the record. Learn to be as consistent in your charting as you have learned to be consistent when taking and recording patient vital signs. Just as you have learned to perform head to toe assessments or address the "ABCs" of a patient in crisis, you can establish a method to record your care in the patient's record.

It is in the standardization of the documentation and the selective use of words to describe events that prudent documentation habits reside. Learn a format and use objective words to relate all pertinent events associated with the patient's care. That is your goal in documentation.

BOX 8.14

Pertinent Negatives

The less evident physical symptoms are difficult to collect and correlate to a patient history. Aspects of the assessment may even be considered a "negative finding." All elements of the patient assessment are valid, but not all are considered relative and pertinent to the patient's complaint. Assessment findings can be either negative or positive, with the negative findings sometimes being considered irrelevant to the current complaint. There are many times when a negative finding may in fact be relevant and pertinent to the patient's initial complaint or to the progression of the patient's illness. For instance, a patient may complain of dizziness and "feeling faint" at the same time his left hand lost strength and abilities in fine motor control. If upon later assessment the patient's grip and strength returned to his left hand, the "finding" for sensory and motor deficit would be considered "negative," but the change in the progression of the patient's illness is considered extremely relevant and pertinent. Another example would be of a change, generally toward an improvement, in a patient's pain response. Improvements in pain may indicate another continued negative finding, but one relevant to the patient's condition. Acknowledging pertinent negatives to defend assessments and interventions that you perform and document cannot be overemphasized. Learn to discriminate among data for that which most specifically relates to the patient's condition or complaint. Just because an assessment is negative does not necessarily mean it isn't relevant to the patient's condition. If a patient has stated that a symptom is absent and there are no objective data to contradict the patient's statement the nurse's choice of action is justified. If neither the absence of a significant factor nor the clearly objective data is recorded it will likely be regarded as overlooked.

Avoiding Omitted Data

Follow a set format for physical assessment and charting like that of taking and recording patient vital signs. This will help you to decrease the potential for error because your charting has a set format with which to record aspects of patient care; you are less likely to omit data when documenting systematically.

There are many patient events in which an "occurrence" mandates documentation. For example, patient falls, medication errors, elopements, use of behavior modifiers (restraints), conscious sedation administration, verbal or telephone physician orders, presence of IV therapy, or unexpected outcomes from therapy all require specific and specialized charting. Samples for charting such events are included at the end of the chapter.

Remember, the nurse is the patient's advocate and has a licensed duty to protect patients from undue harm. If an adverse patient event occurs or your patient suffers an unexpected and negative outcome, you need to know your facility's policy for recording and reporting such occurrences. You are not excused from laws that govern practice; your documentation of such events will matter.

Nurses are expected to intercede on the behalf of the patient to ensure that they are fully informed and able to make reasonable and informed choices. When an unexpected or adverse event occurs, it is expected that nurses respond appropriately and in accordance with standards for care. Documentation in such events must be in conjunction with the facility's defined policy in order for a nurse to defend that he or she acted according to standard.

To learn more effective documentation strategies it is necessary to be knowledgeable about the facility's policies and procedures. Without a thorough familiarity of facility policy, a nurse may unwittingly submit documentation that contributes to a perception of negligence or malpractice. Your documentation will matter.

The more consistent a nurse can be in using a style and format for charting, the better capable he or she is in selecting discriminating and descriptive language for charting. Take the example of the ordinary and routine recording of patient vital signs. Nurses almost unanimously note vital signs in the order of temperature, pulse, respirations, and blood pressure. Why? Because nurses learn how to take vital signs in a certain order and documentation standards conform with the learned order.

It is a good habit to learn to chart the status of IVs, the response to medications, a patient's intake and output in the same manner each time, no matter for which patient you are caring. Only then can a nurse begin to look at the language selections he or she is making. What words a nurse actually uses to note the status of the IV, the response to a medication, or the quality, character, and amount of that intake or output do matter and can make a critical difference if legal review takes place.

A nurse has to learn to discriminate before better word selection can occur. Formatting what you put into the patient record in a consistent manner positions you to improve your choice of words. In Chapters 2 and 3, you learned a format for performing a patient assessment and collecting data related to that assessment. If a nurse can learn to take vital signs or perform assessments in a prescribed order, then that same nurse can also learn to develop a means to document in a prescribed order. Nurses benefit through conforming to a routine when charting standardized assessments or procedures. As in physical assessment or history collecting process, use of a familiar format will help to improve proficiency in your personal charting practices.

REIMBURSEMENT

The last element of the documentation model relates the business end of health care, to the financial matters of the patient's care. A well-documented patient chart can reduce many problems and unnecessary impact on the health care system. Charting entries must precisely mirror services provided. Medicare and HCFA regulations are very specific as to language that must appear in the patient's record related to reimbursement, and nurses are key contributors to the patient record.

A key component is the necessity to document the patient's primary complaint and history of that complaint. In many settings a nurse interviews the patient for their chief complaint and history of the present illness (HPI). A review of systems (ROS) and personal and social history (P/SH) may also be discussed with the patient at the time of the HPI. The manner and thoroughness with which a nurse documents the HPI, ROS and P/SH will affect what the patient is charged for their services.

Physician and health care facility reimbursement "tracks" are not one and the same, though regulations for reimbursement generally apply equally to both physician and facility. Documentation is directly connected with monetary reimbursement. More complete documentation can result in higher reimbursements. However, physician and facility charges must be accurate and in accordance to regulations.

There are also branches of the government and Medicare dedicated to protecting payer rights and interests. Their responsibility is to determine medical necessity and match payment with event. In all such cases the source for information related to the event is the patient's medical record.

In the astronomical finances of today's health care environment, it is equally important to attend to the paperwork of nursing. Because of the potential effect on reimbursement and to reduce undue financial burden on the patient, nurses must learn to take the time to document in a concise, specific format. Review charting entries with a discriminating eye. By using basic rules for good habits of documentation, a nurse can make a difference. Nursing documentation has a decided impact on quality, as well as the legal and financial aspects of the patient's care.

Answer Guide

Exercise 8.1

1. illness
   Common: sickness
   Technical: abnormal process which interrupts or diminishes a person's functioning

2. injury
   Common: wound or damage; injustice
   Technical: any environmental interruption in a person's ability to adapt or defend state of well-being

3. intervention
   Common: coming between or interference
   Technical: action to alter or modify a process

4. elopement
   Common: run away to get married
   Technical: patient who leaves against medical recommendation or secretly

5. force
   Common: strength or power; compel or inflict against resistance; large group
   Technical: to introduce food through tube to one unwilling or unable to eat

6. integrity
   Common: honesty; strict values
   Technical: soundness of structure, unimpaired

7. compensation
   Common: reimbursement
   Technical: counterbalance; adjustment for defect

8. abandonment
   Common: desert
   Technical: not fulfilling obligation toward patient

9. scope
   Common: the range of action or thought
   Technical: instrument for viewing or listening; a range setting practice parameters

10. standard
    Common: flags or emblem; criterion
    Technical: minimum level used for basis of comparison

11. insult
    Common: derogatory reference to another or to self
    Technical: break in integrity; traumatic event

SAMPLE CHARTING

INTAKE AND OUTPUT

	DATE	2/25/99																						
		11-7	7-3	3-11	24° TOT	11-7	7-3	3-11	24° TOT	11-7	7-3	3-11	24° TOT	11-7	7-3	3-11	24° TOT	11-7	7-3	3-11	24° TOT
I N T A K E	ORAL	100cc	550cc	350cc	1000cc																
	NG (WATER FEEDING)	N/A	N/A	N/A	N/A																
	IV	200cc	200cc	200cc	600cc																
	BLOOD	N/A	N/A	N/A	N/A																
	8 HOUR TOTALS	300cc	750cc	550cc	■				■				■				■				■
	24 HOUR TOTALS	1600cc INTAKE																			
O U T P U T	24 HOUR TOTALS																				
	URINE	50cc	200cc	N/A	250cc																
	CATHETER	N/A	N/A	1200cc	1200cc																
	DRAIN	N/A	N/A	N/A	N/A																
	GASTRIC SUCTION	N/A	N/A	N/A	N/A																
	EMESIS	50cc x̄I	Ø	150cc x̄II	200cc																
	BLOOD	N/A	N/A	N/A	N/A																
	BM / GUIAC	Ī ⊖	Ø	Ø	Ī																
	SPECIMEN SENT TO LAB																				
	8 HOUR TOTALS	100cc	200cc	1350cc	■				■				■				■				■
	SPECIFIC GRAVITY	N/A	N/A	N/A	N/A																
	WEIGHT	148lbs ——→																			
	HEIGHT	5'6" ——→																			
		BKFST	LUNCH	DINNER		BKFST	LUNCH	DINNER		BKFST	LUNCH	DINNER		BKFST	LUNCH	DINNER		BKFST	LUNCH	DINNER	
	% OF DIET EATEN	70%	90%	100%																	

INTAKE AND OUTPUT

IMPRINT AREA

Doe, J

1 TOTAL I & O ONE HOUR BEFORE END OF SHIFT.
2 NIGHT SHIFT COMPLETE PREVIOUS 24 HOUR TOTAL I & O.

GRAPHIC RECORD

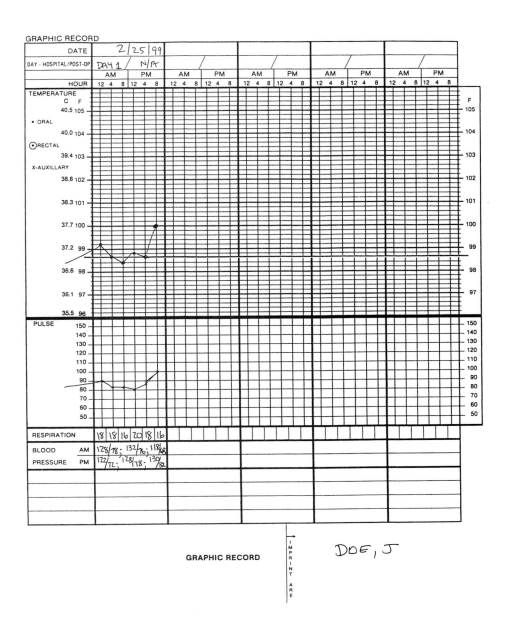

GRAPHIC RECORD

DOE, J

	FLOOR	OR
1. ID Band Checked with Chart by:	DL	
2. A. Consent for Surgery: . . . . Photography	DL	
B. Verify Surgical Procedure c Patient (i.e. correct limb, correct eye) ☒Yes ☐ No	DL	
C. Sterilization Consent: . . . . ☐ Hospital & Government	N/A	
3. A. Allergies (State if known): NONE KNOWN		
B. NPO ☒ Since (What time) 2130	DL	
4. Lab Reports		
A. CBC	DL	
B. Urinalysis	DL	
C. PT/PTT	N/A	
D. Pregnancy Test	N/A	
E. Other	LYTES	
5. Blood Available (Armband Checked) ☐	N/A	
Type and Screen	N/A	
Type and Crossmatch	N/A	
Number of Units Packed Cells	N/A	
6. Chest X-Ray Report (At the discretion of surgeon or Anesthesiologist or if hx. of heart/lung disease)	DL	
7. EKG	DL	
Read: ☒Yes ☐ No (Required 72 hours prior to surgery in patients with positive cardiopulmonary or hypertensive or diuretic indications.)	DL	
8. History and Physical	DL	
9. Old Chart	DL	
10. MAR with Chart: ☒Yes ☐ No		
11. Rand Card with Chart: ☐ Yes ☒No		
12. Addressograph stamp c chart: ☒Yes ☐ No		

13. Prosthesis and Valuables	Removed	Left In	Other	N/A	Explain
(Dentures) Bridges, or Caps:	✓				UPPER/LOWER
Artificial Eyes L - R:				✗	
Artificial Limbs L - R:				✗	
Contact Lens (Glasses:)	✓				
(Ring) Watch, Med/Chain:			✓		TAPED
Wallet:	✓				TO FAMILY
Other:					

14. Surgical Prep: ☐ Yes ☐ No

Signature: _____

Date/Time: _____

15. Vital Signs Pre-Op: T: 98²(c) - 84 (REG.) -16; 108/70

16. Voided: ☒Yes ☐ No Time 0430

Catheter: ☐ Yes ☒No

17. Cap, Gown and Blanket on: ☒Yes ☐ No

18. Pre-Op Teaching:

☒ Verbal

☐ Film

19. Verify understanding of PCA:

☐ Yes

☐ No

☒ N/A

20. Verify understanding of Critical Care (If appropriate):

☐ Yes

☐ No

☒ N/A

21. ☒English ☐ Spanish ☐ Other

Signature of Translator _____

22. Comments: _____

_____

_____

_____

_____

_____

_____

_____

_____

D. Lewis , RN E.D. 0500 2/25/99

Signature of RN/LVN/CNA   (Unit)   Time/Date

_____

Signature of RN/LVN   (Surgery)   Time/Date

Arrival in O.R. (time)

_____

Signature - Transported by

SURGICAL
CHECK
LIST

IMPRINT AREA ►

DOE, J

FORM PVP S426 - STK (4/92)

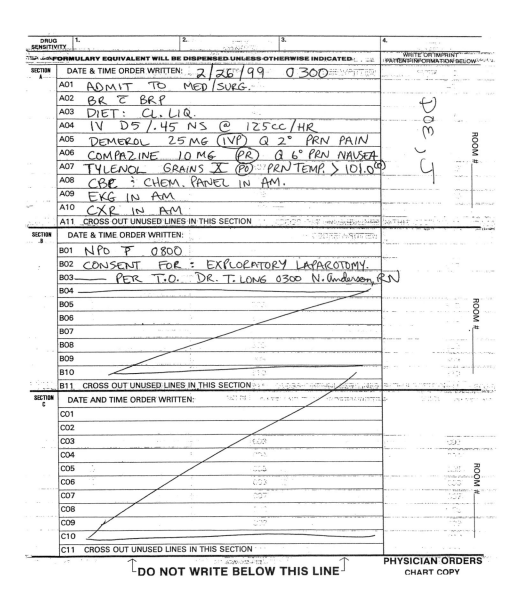

DRUG SENSITIVITY	1.		2.	3.		4.	
	FORMULARY EQUIVALENT WILL BE DISPENSED UNLESS OTHERWISE INDICATED					WRITE OR IMPRINT PATIENT INFORMATION BELOW	

SECTION A — DATE & TIME ORDER WRITTEN: 2/26/99   0300

A01	ADMIT TO MED/SURG.
A02	BR c̄ BRP
A03	DIET: CL. LIQ.
A04	IV D5/.45 NS @ 125CC/HR
A05	DEMEROL 25 MG (IVP) Q 2° PRN PAIN
A06	COMPAZINE 10 MG (PR) Q 6° PRN NAUSEA
A07	TYLENOL GRAINS X (PO) PRN TEMP. > 101.0°
A08	CBC c̄ CHEM. PANEL IN AM.
A09	EKG IN AM
A10	CXR IN AM
A11	CROSS OUT UNUSED LINES IN THIS SECTION

SECTION B — DATE & TIME ORDER WRITTEN:

B01	NPO p̄ 0800
B02	CONSENT FOR : EXPLORATORY LAPAROTOMY.
B03	—— PER T.O. DR. T. LONG 0300 N. Anderson, RN
B04	
B05	
B06	
B07	
B08	
B09	
B10	
B11	CROSS OUT UNUSED LINES IN THIS SECTION

SECTION C — DATE AND TIME ORDER WRITTEN:

C01	
C02	
C03	
C04	
C05	
C06	
C07	
C08	
C09	
C10	
C11	CROSS OUT UNUSED LINES IN THIS SECTION

ROOM #

⌐DO NOT WRITE BELOW THIS LINE⌐

PHYSICIAN ORDERS
CHART COPY

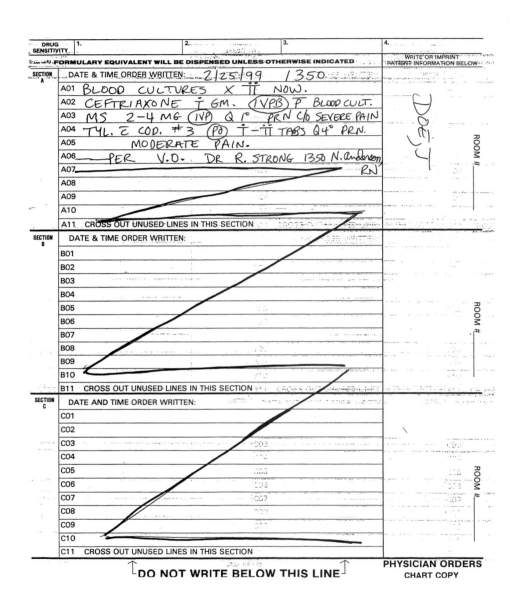

| DRUG SENSITIVITY | 1. | | 2. | | 3. | | 4. | WRITE OR IMPRINT PATIENT INFORMATION BELOW |

FORMULARY EQUIVALENT WILL BE DISPENSED UNLESS OTHERWISE INDICATED

SECTION A

DATE & TIME ORDER WRITTEN: 2/25/99 1350

A01	BLOOD CULTURES X II̅ NOW.
A02	CEFTRIAXONE ī GM. (IVPB) p̄ BLOOD CULT.
A03	MS 2-4 MG (IVP) Q I° PRN C/O SEVERE PAIN
A04	TYL. c̄ COD. #3 (PO) ī-II̅ TABS Q4° PRN.
A05	MODERATE PAIN.
A06	PER V.O. DR R. STRONG 1350 N. Anderson
A07	RN
A08	
A09	
A10	
A11	CROSS OUT UNUSED LINES IN THIS SECTION

SECTION B

DATE & TIME ORDER WRITTEN:

B01	
B02	
B03	
B04	
B05	
B06	
B07	
B08	
B09	
B10	
B11	CROSS OUT UNUSED LINES IN THIS SECTION

SECTION C

DATE AND TIME ORDER WRITTEN:

C01	
C02	
C03	
C04	
C05	
C06	
C07	
C08	
C09	
C10	
C11	CROSS OUT UNUSED LINES IN THIS SECTION

↑ DO NOT WRITE BELOW THIS LINE ↑

PHYSICIAN ORDERS
CHART COPY

ROOM #

DATE	CONCERN	PROGRESS NOTES PAGE NO.
2/25/99		PT. c̄ c/o ABDOMINAL "DISCOMFORT", "8 OF 10", "HOT
0825		FEELING". NON-RADIATING, CONTINUOS x 30 MIN.
		NOW ↑INGLY WORSE. Ø ↑ IN COMPLAINTS c̄ DEEP
		INSPIRATION OR ACTIVITY. STATES "SITTING STRAIGHT
		UP HELPS". ———————————————— N. Anderson, RN
0835		DEMEROL 75MG / VISTARIL 50MG IM (RUOQ). ——— N. Anderson RN
0850		PT. STATES "PAIN IS MUCH BETTER NOW". RATES PAIN
		"4 OF 10" NOW. ABLE TO TURN TO SIDE s̄ ACUTE COMPLAINT.
		TOL. SIPS FLUIDS s̄ NAUSEA. RESPONSIVE APPROPRIATELY
		TO VERBAL. SKIN W/D. ——————————— N. Anderson, RN

DOE, J

CLIENT NAME

PROGRESS NOTES

DATE	CONCERN	PROGRESS NOTES	PAGE NO.
2/25/99 0800		IV SITE TO (RT) HAND c̄ 20G. CATH. INTACT. Ø S+S REDNESS, SWELLING, Ø c/o TENDERNESS TO PALP. Ø S+S DRAINAGE NOTED. IV #2 NS @ TKO. DRSG. DRY AND INTACT. —— N. Anderson, RN	
2/25/99 1000		IV DRSG. Δ'D. SITE INTACT s̄ S+S REDNESS OR SWELLING. PT. c/o "SL. TENDERNESS" TO PALP. Ø DRAINAGE NOTED. #20G. CATH. INTACT. IV#2 INFUSING AS ORDERED. —— N. Anderson, RN	
2/25/99 1100		IV#2 c̄ REDNESS & TENDERNESS @ SITE. IV DC'D, CATH. INTACT. IV RESTARTED (LT) HAND c̄ 22G. CATH., 1ST ATTEMPT. IV#2 NS @ TKO —————————— N. Anderson, RN	

DOE, J

CLIENT NAME

PROGRESS NOTES

DATE	CONCERN	PROGRESS NOTES PAGE NO.
2/25/99		DR. SPOCK IN FOR EVAL, OK FOR DISCHARGE HOME
1100AM		c̄ PARENTS. CHILD CON'T PLAYFUL, INTERACTIVE c̄
		MOTHER. ALERT TO STIMULUS AND ACTIVITY. CHILD
		c̄ AGE-APPROPRIATE BEHAVIORS AND RESPONSES. SKIN
		W/D/PINK, RESPIRATIONS EVEN c̄ Ø S+S RESP. DISTRESS,
		INFREQ. COUGH, NON-PRODUCTIVE @ THIS TIME /OBSERVA-
		TION. DISCHARGE INSTRUCTIONS RE. MEDS, FLUIDS,
		TYLENOL USAGE AND PMD F/U IF Ø IMPROVED IN
		2-3 DAYS. CHILD AMBULATORY ON DISCH. HOME c̄
		MOTHER —————————————————— N. Anderson, RN

DOE, J

CLIENT NAME

PROGRESS NOTES

DATE	CONCERN	PROGRESS NOTES	PAGE NO.
2/27/99 0720		PT. FOUND ON FLOOR, SUPINE BY SIDE OF BED. PT. STATING "I DON'T KNOW HOW THIS HAPPENED, I WAS TRYING TO GO TO THE BATHROOM." IV NS LOCK INTACT TO (R) FOREARM. 4 SIDERAILS IN "UP" POSITION, BED IN "LOW" HEIGHT. PT. ALERT TO PLACE, PERS BUT UNABLE TO RECALL DATE/TIME. SKIN W/D/P. Ø OBVIOUS WOUNDS OR BLEEDING NOTED @ THIS TIME PT STATES "I'M OK" ON REQUEST c̄ C/O "I FEEL FOOLISH". RETD TO BED c̄ ASSIST OF -2- STAFF. DR DOUGLASS NOTIFIED VIA PHONE. VS: 97⁸⁶⁽⁰⁾ 88-20; 102/60 IN LYING SUPINE POSITION. NS LOCK SITE INTACT, Ø SWELLING, REDNESS OR TENDERNES NOTED. LUNGS CTA. SIDERAILS REMAIN UP.———N.Anderson	
0745		DR DOUGLASS NOTIFIED RE. PT. ↑'INGLY AGGITATED CONDITION. SKIN W/D/PINK. AP: 92, RR: 20 c̄ RESP. EVEN, EQUAL @ REST. PT. CONSOLABLE c̄ STAFF VERBA INTERVENTION BUT RETURNS TO RESTLESS AND STATE "I NEED TO GET OUT OF HERE RIGHT NOW". LUNGS REMAIN CLEAR BILAT. Ø S+S RESP. DISTRESS c̄ AGGITATION. STAFF PRESENT c̄ PT.@ BEDSIDE—N.Anderson	
0755		BEHAVIOR MODIFIERS (RESTRAINTS) TO 4 EXTREMITY PER MD T.O. PT. TOL. MODIFIERS s̄ DISTRESS, STATES "ARE THESE NECESSARY?". CALMS c̄ STAFF VERBAL ORIENTATION TO TIME, PLACE, PERSON FAMILY NOTIFIED RE. PT. Δ' IN STATUS, DGHTR. TO COME IN THIS AM. PT. SETTLES TO RESTING QUIET c̄ Ø ACUTE Δ'S. SIDERAILS "UP" POSITION. ⊕ CMS TO HANDS/FEET BILAT. LUNGS CONT CLEAR. PERIF ERAL PERFUSION INTACT. PT. OFFERED URINAL BUT DENIES NEED TO VOID.———N. Anderson, R	
0810		CMS CHECKED, CONT EQUAL TO ~~ALL 4 SIDES~~(NA) FOUR ^MISTAKEN ENTRY EXTREMITIES. PT. c̄ Ø ACUTE Δ'S OR COMPLAINTS NOTED. REMAINS CONFUSED TO TIME, REORIENTS EASILY—N. Anderse	

DOE, J

TIME	VITAL SIGNS	I.V.s AND MEDICATIONS	NURSE NOTES/SIGNATURE	INIT
1100			PT. RESTING QUIETLY IN BED. OFFERS Ø COMPLAINTS. STATES IS "ANXIOUS FOR THE DOCTOR TO GET HERE". ———— N. Anderson RN	
1130	T: 97⁸-72-16 118/74 O₂ SAT: 99% (RA)		Ø ACUTE Δ'S IN PT. CONDITION NOTED. ASKS "IS THE DOCTOR HERE YET? I WANT TO SEE HIM RIGHT AWAY". SKIN W/D, RESPIRATIONS EVEN c̄ Ø DISTRESS NOTED ON PT. EFFORT OR EXERTION—N. Anderson, RN	
1220			PT. NOTED NOT IN ROOM WHEN CHECKED. SUPERVISOR/SECURITY NOTIFIED. PT. GOWN ON BED, PT. CLOTHING NOT IN CLOSET. PT. IN BED "A" STATES PT. PUT ON STREET CLOTHES AND SAID "I'M OUTTA HERE, I CAN'T WAIT FOR THAT DOCTOR ANY LONGER. I'M SUPPOSED TO GO HOME TODAY AND I AM." PMD CONTACTED AS TO PT. AMA. LOCAL PD CONTACTED BY HOUSE SUPERVISOR. ———— N. Anderson, RN	

TOTAL INTAKE _____ cc	TOTAL OUTPUT _____ cc	DISPOSITION OF CLOTHES AND VALUABLES:
CLOTHING:	VALUABLES:	
		GIVEN TO:
		RELATIONSHIP:
		NURSE SIG.:

PAGE 2

→ IMPRINT AREA →

DOE, J

CHAPTER 9

Putting It Together for Practical Use

It is now time to review the key concepts that have been presented in this book. As you review each of these points make notations of those you feel need further review. Documentation is similar to other nursing functions in that repetition aids in gaining proficiency. As you have learned thus far, repeating any task correctly each and every time allows you to form good habits that become automatic in practice.

Chapter 1 introduced you to this text. You were invited to learn the vocabulary and format techniques used in improving documentation. You may review this chapter and decide if the text offers further choices that serve to enhance what has been covered in subsequent chapters. It explains how the authors intended the book to be used for the best results. It also allows you to make decisions about your personal use of the text.

Students usually recognize the study style that suits them best. For instance, a student may decide to use the interactive exercises as an adjunct to the text or to copy exercises from the text as "carry along" materials in clinical settings. The text may be read before doing interactive exercises or may be used concurrently. Some students may decide to use the text or computer versions exclusively. This is not recommended, because the interactive exercises are clarified by the text narrative and provide practice for the student in a graded format. The material presented is intended to be used in any way to improve the student's ability to chart and give report in the best and most effective way possible.

BOX 9.1

Key Concepts: Chapter 2

Common Terms, Unfamiliar Definitions

Learning the Language

Patient Care Impact

Spelling

Handwriting

Shorthand, Abbreviations, Pictures

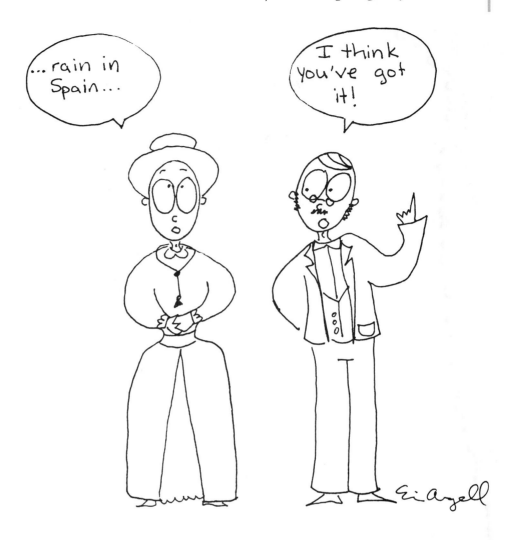

COMMON TERMS, UNFAMILIAR DEFINITIONS

The introduction of common terms, or words, that have more technical meanings stands as self-explanatory. The use of language is fluid. By the time this text is published there will likely be new techniques used in medicine and nursing that "borrow" words from the common use or from other disciplines and incorporate those words into medical usage.

Certainly the use of computers at the bedside opens the door to the possibility of charting on-line using voice technology or keyboards. Centralized documentation, eliminating the use of written charting, has introduced "shadow" charting, the practice by nurses and medical doctors of keeping private charts as they believe necessary. These hidden charts are the direct result of changes in documentation methods and the need to alter the use of paper charting. So get ready to start hearing requests for "hard copy," and for blending technical computer language into the health care system.

Students may create their own word lists generated from the clinical setting. Individual facilities in each region of the country adopt idiosyncratic use of language. This practice may create problems if inconsistent with acceptable procedure by payers such as insurance companies and public reimbursement programs. If nurses note the inclusion of region-specific language and/or abbreviations, these need to be included in the setting's lists of acceptable terms.

A standard needs to be adopted and adhered to that justifies use of forms, words, and style as acceptable within the clinic itself, and is appropriate for legal and cost reimbursement purposes.

Public programs such as Medicare and Medicaid may establish their own guidelines for documentation that are limited to including only widely accepted terminology. They also introduce their language into the mix. For example, in cost-justifying some home health care visits, "housebound" status of the patient must be included in the documentation. Medicare is not referring to "snow days." They intended that the patient meet a specific criteria, that of limited mobility that does not allow them to independently visit a provider. Consequently the provider offers care in the home.

LEARNING THE LANGUAGE

Student nurses may feel that they are learning medical terminology through immersion, a respected technique for learning languages. While this does work eventually, as this text emphasizes, learning words individually and in context supports the learning process.

Nursing programs are continually evolving in order to offer their students complete and current theory and skills content. Because these programs are obligated to fulfill their teaching obligations and to remain within a set number of required units, this often means that the curriculum reflects the faculty's priorities. Documentation skills may be linked to specific skills taught in the lab or, in some cases, taught only "as needed" in the clinical setting. Instructors may even rationalize minimal instruction in documentation due to the increased use of preprinted forms to replace narrative charting. The clinical and legal value of narrative charting that is clear and precise does not diminish because we, as teachers, have limited time.

In reviewing Chapter 2, it is up to the student to determine the impact that learning correct language and format will have on his or her personal practice. They can revisit the exercises that demonstrate how language can lead to misinterpretation of actual and factual data. We believe that the time spent by nurses in developing good documentation habits reflects their professionalism and their practice.

PATIENT CARE IMPACT

Data from nursing staff documentation potentially affect patient care for better or for worse. Be mindful that nursing notes can make a significant difference to the patient. On this key concept the text has based the need to be objective, to quantify descriptors, to avoid bias, and to spell correctly.

Correct spelling is not a frivolous matter when weighed against the potential consequences. Take the time to reread the examples of spelling errors and how the error can change the nature of the patient's care. Consider the damage possible if drugs are misspelled. And remember that medical staff might also be responsible for spelling errors. Should you read an order for a drug, especially one that is spelled like another very different drug, and if the written dosage is inconsistent with a usual dosage for that drug, call the physician.

When spelling creates uncertainty regarding patient orders, it is always appropriate to confirm the order with the physician. It is also true that the provider might be prickly about being misunderstood or verified. The medical provider's feelings need to be secondary to the appropriate and clear understanding of written orders. If error related to unclear writing or poor spelling leads to a patient problem, or even to an event with no adverse outcome, nurses can be sure that the provider will be quick to say, "You should have called."

JUDICIOUS USE OF SYMBOLS

Learn to use symbols that replace words in the same way that you use common abbreviations. Use them judiciously, since the purpose of the symbols is to enhance clarity, not to add confusion. Individual clinical settings may use shorthand techniques that are narrowly targeted to specialties. When orienting, ask about this practice. It is also appropriate to ask about abbreviations or symbols to which you are introduced during a rotation. Don't be embarrassed about asking. It might alert the staff that they are also unclear about a provider's intent.

The authors have had the experience of asking, with a student, about the meaning of an abbreviation written by a physician. We were unable to find a nurse who knew what the abbreviation meant. This problem highlights the danger of documentation that is not clear or common in a particular setting. If the caregivers cannot understand the note, it does not serve to improve patient care. If the data in the note are critical it can endanger the patient.

The message to take away is to use clearly understood symbols and not to be afraid to ask questions about symbols or abbreviations that are not in your current vocabulary.

WRITING AND SPELLING

There is no justification for patient care errors that could have been prevented by clear documentation or rechecking an order that was unclear. All health providers are being reminded that deadly mistakes can be avoided by taking precautions to write clearly and spell correctly. With the increased use of computers at the bedside and electronic charting, the handwriting issues may be solved with the use of up-to-date equipment. It is still unclear how spelling errors will be managed, because similar drug names and similar words depend on accurate human input.

Computers programmed to correct spelling will not solve this problem, because software cannot decide which word was intended. The problem could be exacerbated by complacent care team members. Computers will never replace critical thinking skills.

BOX 9.2

Key Concepts: Chapter 3

Documentation Format
Order and Organization

DOCUMENTATION FORMAT

The primary purpose of Chapter 3 is to provide nurses with acceptable charting formats that organize data into logical order. In a sense, the key concept is the whole of the information presented, because we believe that the use of a set and consistent format is instrumental in providing good care as well as recording the data related to care.

The key concept focuses on teaching nurses to discipline their thinking process by collecting data in a specific order, prioritizing their recorded note to ensure that critical data are not overlooked, and by clearly stating all significant information as well as related relevant data.

The formats presented are those most commonly taught in medical and nursing programs and are consistent with the formats preferred by insurance providers, both private and public. These are also in accord with the head-to-toe format commonly used in physical assessment. It is our belief that expertise in organization allows the nurse an advantage; it is easier to remember a missing element when one is accustomed to following a repetitive routine than it is if one is accustomed to a less organized method of examination.

It is not the intention of this text to minimize the value of any other format used in a specific setting. There is, however, the question of using printed checklists exclusively and disallowing appropriate attention to narrative charting. While it is true that checklists are provided to eliminate subjective and inaccurate characterization of a patient's status, they are necessarily limited to language that may not appropriately describe specific data.

A mental exercise that helps to emphasize this point is one to which student nurses may easily relate. Students are given the opportunity to evaluate individual classes for the content and quality of instruction. The offered choices do not always portray the students' true feelings about either.

For instance, the student may like a specific instructor but be unimpressed by her performance in presenting some or all of the material in a class. Or they may have enjoyed the material presented but felt that the text had little or no relevance as support material. If their choices are limited to "excellent, good, fair, or poor" they may feel that "fair" is too low a value, or just does not characterize the class appropriately. So they may skew the evaluation upward, even though they don't agree. The "good" evaluation may result in the faculty's continuing to use a text that is mismatched with a particular class.

This type of confusion affects the subsequent students enrolled in the class. If you apply the analogy to a patient, there is far greater impact than that on the students. If a patient's response to a medication or treatment is mischaracterized, the complete course of care may be altered. There is always the risk of misunderstanding or miscommunication. If communication error is compounded because nurses are compelled to use a checklist exclusively, patient care outcomes may be affected adversely.

Prioritization, relevancy, organization and brevity, accuracy, and efficiency are the key concepts stressed for narrative charting that is accurate and efficient. We choose to emphasize these points again in the summary as they are also necessary in care delivery. Since cost efficiency within care settings alter staffing ratios, nurses are forced to become time management experts. Often they need to choose what care must be given "now" and delay or delegate less necessary functions. We do not intend to minimize the role of nursing. However, it is often difficult for graduate nurses to adapt to time constraints placed by workload. Tough choices are made daily by nurses, which require judgment and rationale. The nurse who has learned these key elements is at an advantage.

CHARACTERIZING SYMPTOMS

We stress the importance of complete and accurate characterization of a patient's symptom, or complaint. In any format chosen, it is necessary to state the patient's own complaint and all modifiers of that complaint. Even if the patient has misinterpreted the meaning of the symptoms, as with cardiac patients whose chief complaint is gastric distress or heartburn. The descriptors are one of the most important factors in the nurse's assessment note. They are key concepts that are necessary for good practice.

BOX 9.3

Key Concepts: Chapter 4

Syntax, Nursing Notes
Integrating Information
Language That "Implies" Action
Creating the Word Picture

SYNTAX, NURSING NOTES

Understanding syntax assists in organization of thought and action. Dangling modifiers contribute to confusion and miscommunication. There are times that nurses wish to add a descriptor after committing parts of the assessment to the chart. They need to be careful to clarify the importance of the descriptor and be able to alert a team member to the addition. Key, relevant assessment data may affect care. Review this section of Chapter 4 if the concept of syntax is confusing.

The overall review of syntax reminds the nurse that how a note is presented affects the perception of the note by subsequent care team members. If a provider is interrupted prior to reading a complete note, they may never complete the task; hence the importance of prioritization and of brevity. If the information in the beginning of the note is trivial or ancillary to the immediate needs of the patient, the value of the complete note is compromised.

INTEGRATING INFORMATION

Time management skills are basic to nursing practice. Chapter 4 emphasizes the integration of the learning process, which assists the nursing student in minimizing their workload. As the student visualizes the history format and physical assessment pattern in the context of charting, the concept of integration becomes clear. Repetition of learned skills makes more sense as the patterns for organizing each skill are nearly identical.

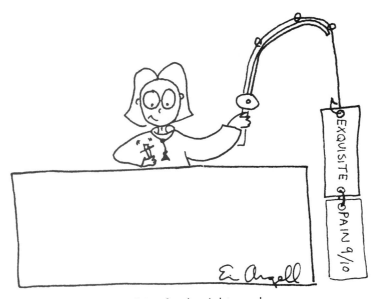

Fishing for the right word

Repetition, or rote, learning methods are sometimes viewed as too concrete or methodical to have broad value. In fact, all learning techniques that encourage better retention of information and subsequently minimize the risk of error or omission by a caregiver are valuable.

To repeat, review the charting format with the emphasis on consistency and compare this with the CHH and the head-to-toe physical assessment. The relationship among these allows you to be efficient in data collection as well as being thorough and specific.

LANGUAGE THAT "IMPLIES" ACTION

One of the primary reasons that nursing units run efficiently and that team efforts by providers, such as seen in operating rooms, or in doing procedures, is the nurse's ability to anticipate what is necessary in delivering care. On a small scale, each nurse must gather appropriate equipment to change a dressing or insert a catheter without making several trips to the supply closet or without having to interrupt a procedure to retrieve forgotten items.

In a broader context, the exercises that were offered for understanding this key concept showed you how you can walk through a care plan and be prepared for a nursing action just by anticipating need based on a single word. Students may have heard this referred to as "thinking like a nurse." *It is actually using language in context with the experience gained through practice.* In medical school it is said of procedures that the student sees one, does one, then teaches one. In nursing practice, this type of rapid learning also occurs. After the nurse observes the appropriate response to an event he or she should review the process and be prepared for a subsequent like experience.

In some cases, such as individual procedures performed, cards are kept that indicate the preferences of individual providers. This works well if the procedure is planned in advanced and the nurse has opportunity to prepare. In emergency or rapidly changing situations, however, nurses need to prepare and respond based on key words, knowledge of the usual response, and the supplies and personnel most likely necessary and available. Each facility will have some differences in their expected response to specific events. Nurses should have a rationale to justify their response. This rationale is often based on the same key language that generated the response in the first place.

CREATING THE WORD PICTURE

This key concept is simple but not easy. It emphasizes that the words used in documentation necessarily must describe as accurately as possible the patient, the problem, and the contributing data related to assessment, intervention, and outcome. Refer once again to the emphasis placed on prioritization, relevance, organization, brevity, and efficiency of language.

The picture of the patient and the problem that you document determines the arrangement of the picture. For example, the primary or immediate problem should be in full focus. Supporting data are either part of the sharply focused issue or are suitable in the background. Data that have peripheral significance should be prominent enough to be noticed but should not be in the spotlight.

Practice your observation skills by looking at a familiar location. Write down what you first notice. Follow up with other details that you remember. Do this each time you see that exact location for several days. There may be a dominant focal point that dominates each time. Or the activity around the location may vary so that each observation has specific, detailed differences.

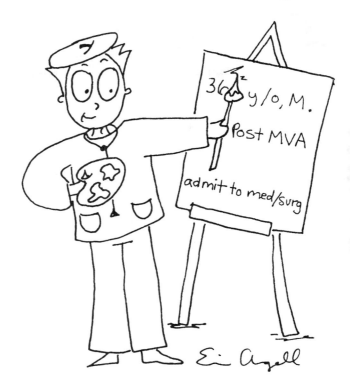

This is similar to what should occur as you document the progress of the patient. Ideally the initial note focuses on the presenting problem, transitions through the recovery period, and concludes with a discharge assessment. As noted earlier, the practice of painting the patient picture is a simple concept but not always easy to accomplish.

BOX 9.4

Key Concepts: Chapter 5

The Difference Between Subjective and Objective Data
Where Do Biases Come From?
Inflammatory Words or Judgment Statements
Value Judgments and Related Language
Nursing Diagnoses: A Factual Data Base

SUBJECTIVE AND OBJECTIVE DATA

The differentiation between objective and subjective data is usually straightforward. The challenge is to document each observation in objective language. Practicing this skill can be fun. You might reinforce your observation skills by doing some group exercises. Those suggested here can be done alone but may be more fun and yield increased information if done in a group.

1. Put on a blindfold. Have a classmate present you with an object that you must describe. Do not name the object, describe what you feel. Your partner can write down the description. An additional challenge would be to share the description with a classmate who did not participate to see if he or she can guess what you described from your note. This is also a good group exercise for critical thinking.

2. Describe odors without using the source name or origin. Words that are commonly used are sour, acrid, sweet, smoky, or burned. Imagine you were experiencing the odor for the first time.
3. Touch objects that have different textures. Describe the object. Share your descriptions with a classmate and see if he or she can match the description to the correct object. Use many types of objects, from fabric to oatmeal.
4. Use music to sharpen your ability to differentiate tone and tempo. Classical music works best but other music is also appropriate. Describe the sounds of various instruments. Describe the tempo or rate. Music has resonance, pitch, depth, and vibration. After you play with music, revisit the heart and lung sound audio aids in the skills lab and describe what you hear.

It is much easier to describe these sensations in subjective terms. The challenge is to create an objective picture with language.

BIAS WORDS AND THEIR ORIGINS

To understand the impact of labeling a patient by using bias words, take a minute to recall words in your own vocabulary that demonstrate your own biases. These words may be said in jest, as put downs, or in fact could be used in a serious manner without thought of the judgment implicit in the language. The best first step in eliminating this type of language from your professional vocabulary is to be aware that it exists. Reflect on the contrast between the actual definition of a bias word and the intent and context of its use. If you find yourself using a bias word, write down the word and the comment in which you used it. Read the comment after a day or two has passed. The comment in written form is likely to sound offensive.

It is helpful for nurses to examine and acknowledge their own biases. We all have them. They come in the form of opinions based on experience or exposure. As nurses we expect to treat all patients with equal respect and care. This is a difficult task if we are unaware that we all have the potential to provide poor care to those who we may fear or by whom we are repulsed. Or, we may give adequate but minimal care.

We also might document subjective issues raised by the patient as less believable or take less care to determine the validity of such complaints. Biases take many forms and can influence nursing practice. Nurses can have bias regarding those who have too little or too much; those who are unemployed; single parents; adolescents involved in violent activity; people of color; those who don't speak English; the undocumented. No group is insulated from bias.

The most effective way to protect your own practice standards from the taint of bias is being aware of personal bias.

INFLAMMATORY WORDS OR JUDGMENT STATEMENTS

No nurse *enjoys* the task of discussing painful subjects with patients. In many cases language that is highly emotional must be used to avoid misleading a patient. For instance a patient in the end stages of renal or liver disease may need to be comforted but also has a right to be informed regarding the gravity of his or her situation. If a nurse is documenting patient teaching with respect to signing a DNR and never used the words "do not resuscitate," the charting should reflect the actual words used with the patient.

Understanding the effect that blunt language has on open communication is important. Language also affects interaction among the staff. A terminal patient may have a primary provider who is unable to accept the "failure" of a patient to respond to treatment. Providers may avoid confronting the severity of the moment with patients and with other providers. They may read a note and react to the use of these trigger words with the same distress as the patient. There are providers who hedge words so successfully that patients will end up asking a nurse what exactly the provider meant.

Situations in which the nurse is unsure about the patient's understanding of the disease process or of a procedure presents ethical and moral issues regarding informed consent. The provider's documented note may conflict with the patient's subjective understanding. Nurses frequently are left with difficult situations that need to be documented carefully and with understanding about the effects of inflammatory language that are impediments to good communication.

VALUE JUDGMENTS

The key concept related to value judgments is simple. The subjective value judgment about a patient does not belong in the chart. Patient care conferences may provide the nurse a place to vent their frustration regarding a particular patient. But the language used in documenting assessment of the patient or of the patient's response to care needs to be as objectively worded as possible.

The key concepts in Chapter 5 are interrelated and affect verbal communication as well as written documentation. The "take home message" is to encourage nurses to do a self-evaluation. Know the biases that you have. Understand that words that trigger highly emotional responses may effectively block communication. Be aware of the impact your subjective comments about a patient may have on his or her care. Know how you can bias others about a patient because the patient has affected you in a negative fashion.

NURSING DIAGNOSES: A FACTUAL DATA BASE

Understanding the syntax of the nursing diagnosis is necessary in learning their use. While some facilities do not use nursing diagnoses in their documentation or patient care plan, it is helpful for nurses to understand the basis for determining each diagnosis. By documenting assessment data that validates the interventions recommended for a nursing diagnosis the nurse justifies the care given. Justification of care affects any review of the nurse's professional standard, either by a hospital quality assurance team, or by a court of law. It also justifies each intervention in the event that the insurance provider questions if an intervention was necessary for the patient.

We do not like to be constantly reminded of the cost of providing care. We do not like to be limited in our ability to provide what we determine to be adequate and necessary care. And, we don't like to do paperwork. This is a conundrum in which we need to limit our complaining about overdocumenting and err on the safe side for the patient.

BOX 9.5
Key Concepts: Chapter Six

Gathering Data
Symptom Descriptors with Associated Words
Putting the Pieces Together

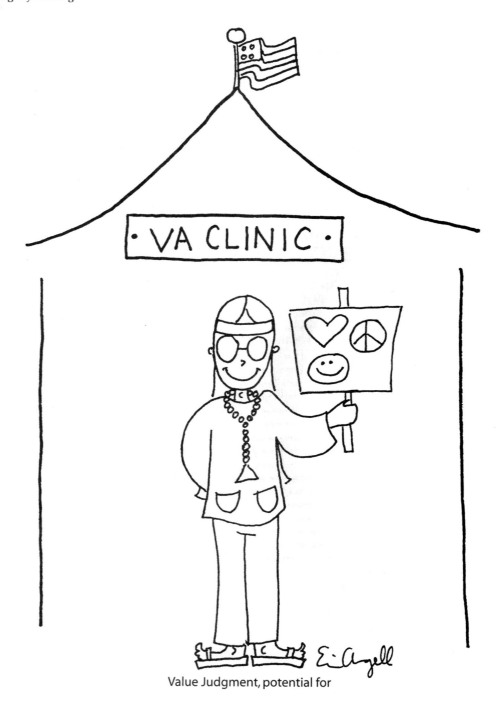

Value Judgment, potential for

GATHERING DATA

Consistency plays a major role in this key concept. If nurses determine the standard by which they personally measure subjective findings and they do not deviate from this standard, their notes will positively affect patient care. This is true even if individual nurses disagree on the meaning of the scale. Individual determinations will never deviate greatly from one another within a standard. The factor that creates the most deviations is the value each nurse gives to the patient's subjective perception.

If the nurse listens to the patient and records the patient's evaluation of a subjective symptom, the nurse's biases will not negatively affect care. For instance, a patient who appears to overstate pain will be supported or not supported by physical assessment and objective findings. A patient who states that medication is not working, but is observed resting quietly or has improved mobility, is not considered unreliable. The nurse clearly documents the objective measurements as well as the patient's perception without passing any judgment. The provider then has the information necessary for making any medication adjustment.

The documentation validates decisions made and supports interventions as being consistent with care standards. Outcomes are also evaluated as objectively as possible using consistent measurable scales.

Patients who are unable to respond are assessed and treated based on objective data alone. However some "objective" data such as those used in the Glasgow coma scale have a subjective component: the individual nurse's baseline understanding. Again, consistency by the individual nurse in evaluating each patient is the key to positive patient impact.

NORMAL: DIFFERENT AMONG INDIVIDUALS

We have all made the comment "Is that normal?" about a physical response or about social or cultural behavior. Many nurses use the term *dysfunctional* interchangeably with *abnormal*. There are differences, and the key is in recognizing a vast range for normal. Some are functional and some not so much. The word dysfunctional can be applied to any system, physical or psychosocial that does not work. It does not function to the betterment of the patient involved.

There are instances when a physical or psychosocial environment deviates from what is considered normal yet is functional for the individual. For instance there are patients with chronic respiratory disease who have oxygen levels that are severely abnormal. Increasing the O2 availability in these patients could be detrimental instead of helpful since it could depress the body's own respiratory mechanism. The patient may also have adapted to the lower oxygen supply. So, this patient's normal is abnormal but functional.

When the nurse charts on this patient, the note cannot read WNL or "within normal limits," even if the patient maintains at the abnormal level. This standard is true for patients who normally have seizures or who routinely have episodes of dyspnea.

The challenge with normally abnormal patients is charting to emphasize change in the patient's status. Deviations that are potentially life-threatening may be overlooked if they are not prioritized in documentation and in verbal report. The developmentally disabled and patients who are unable to communicate are especially vulnerable. The nurse becomes their voice; this is an awesome relationship and an awful responsibility.

EXPERTISE COMES WITH TIME AND PRACTICE

Students may get discouraged if they cannot do a complete and rapid verbal report or if they seem to "take forever" deciding what to write in a patient's chart. Fluid charting takes practice. We emphasize the importance of using a consistent format precisely to assist the student in gaining proficiency through regular practice. Nurses who work in specific areas gain proficiency in that area of expertise. If they change jobs they can apply their knowledge to a different unit as they build their knowledge base and vocabulary.

Students begin with a very small knowledge base. With time and practice they learn the details necessary for good documentation. This process is simplified if they learn to follow a specific format and build a base of good documentation habits.

MAKING GOALS OBJECTIVE

Documentation is a written record that demonstrates compliance with expected course of patient care. Who makes the rules or states the guidelines that demand compliance. This is a tough question that has no easy answer.

As noted in Chapter 6, quality assurance departments are the overseers of care. They require that clear and objective measurable goals be set for the patient. They prefer long-term as well as short-term goals. Students learn to include these in their nursing care plans.

Many facilities have abandoned the use of the care plan, but not the requirement for stated objective goals. Clinical pathways have stated generic goals for the presenting problem. Individual goals may be added, or goals may vary, as patients don't always stay on the path.

Goals that state length of hospital stay and expected outcomes are used by insurance providers to determine if they will accept the stated charges. Nurses are offended, and reasonably so, by the emphasis on cost reimbursement. However, facts are facts. Payors demand documentation that justifies the charges that they are expected to pay. Nurses and other hospital staff command reasonable salaries and are essential employees in care facilities. It is only logical that clear objective documentation is the price we pay for being able to practice nursing, maintain high standards, and be reasonably reimbursed for what we do.

INTUITIVE DATA

This is a key concept that is often overlooked or undervalued. It does not matter if nurses do not agree about the nature of "intuitive" data. It may be a feeling nurses get or the result of cumulative bits of objective data. It should not be ignored but cannot be documented as intuition. The bits and pieces of objective data should be documented as rationale for intuitive actions.

We believe that nurses need not be defensive or embarrassed about this unexplained phenomena. As with other intangible situations that do not lend themselves to easy explanation, intuition by nurses related to patient care remains a mystery.

SYMPTOM DESCRIPTORS

The following cartoons demonstrate the characteristics of a symptom.

BOX 9.6

Key Concepts: Chapter 7

Review of Systems

A. General status	J. Gastrointestinal
B. Skin, hair, nails	K. Urinary tract
C. Eyes	L. Genital
D. Ears	M. Musculoskeletal
E. Nose, sinus	N. Neuro
F. Mouth, throat	O. Endocrine
G. Breasts	P. Hematopoietic
H. Respiratory	Q. Psychological status
I. Cardiovascular	R. OB/GYN

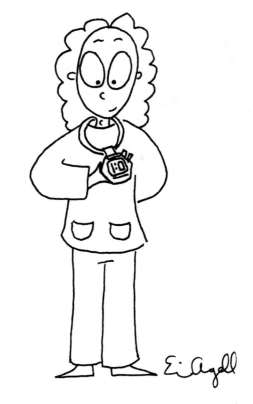

On your mark, get set.....

ONSET

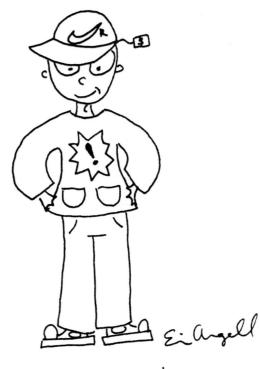

Not again!

QUALITY

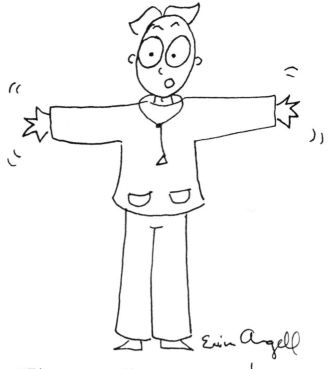

It was this much!

QUANTITY

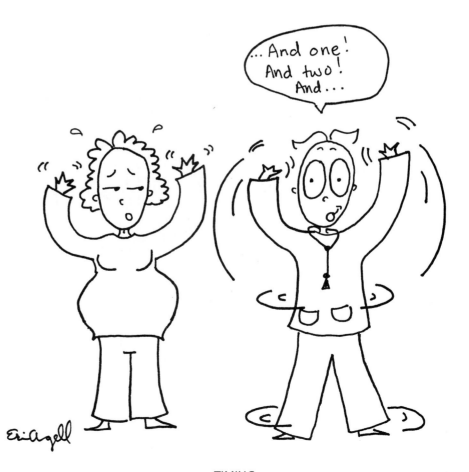

TIMING

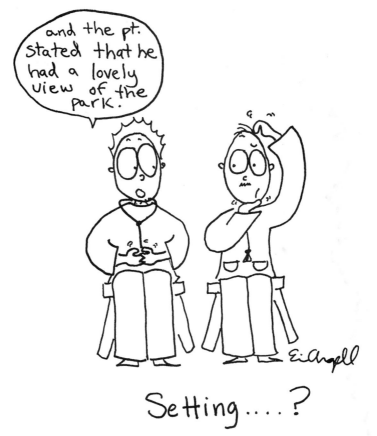

SETTING

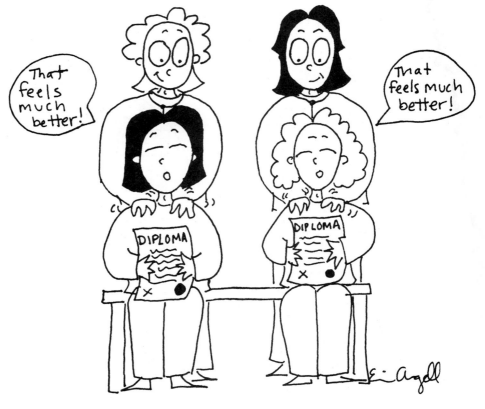

BETTER/WORSE

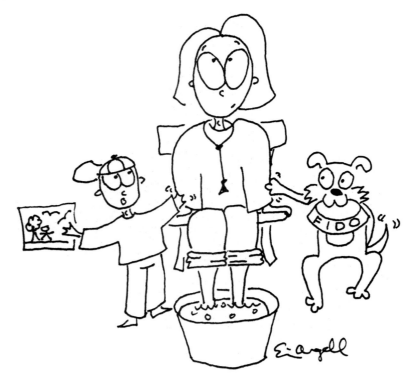

ASSOCIATED MANIFESTATIONS

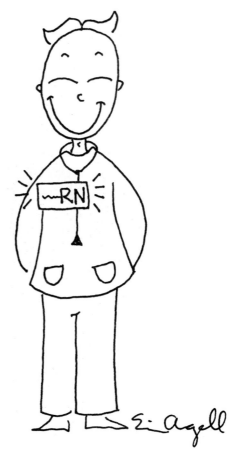

MEANING TO PATIENT I

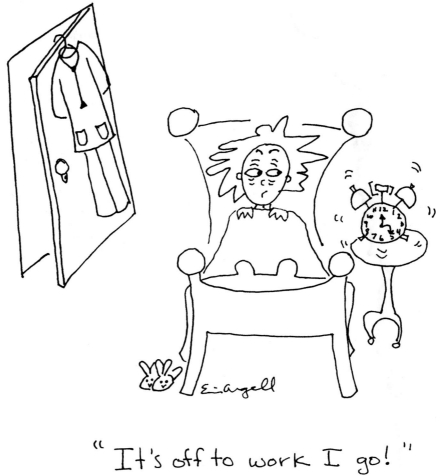

" It's off to work I go! "

MEANING TO PATIENT II

Chapter 7 provides the opportunity to practice charting technique and style. No new key concepts are introduced. All key concepts are implemented. The ROS is once again emphasized as a universal guideline for organization. This chapter helps you practice charting in many different clinical areas. The exercises can be repeated as presented; you may choose to prepare verbal reports. Use this chapter to develop skills and meet individual needs. Demonstrate your strengths and strengthen your weak areas.

It may be helpful to review the case studies and determine how you may have made different choices in charting if some of the information was different. The focus of the case studies is less on process and greater on determining the type of information given and how to actually write the note. However slight variations of the data will affect the prioritization of the information.

You can refer back to the case studies when you have patients with similar stories. It is unlikely the course of the patient's illness will mimic the case study exactly, but when you include a review of similar documentation in your clinical preparation, you reinforce data gathering and recording skills.

Perhaps the primary concept to remember from Chapter 7 is the following: *Expertise in documentation is gained through time and practice.*

> **BOX 9.7**
>
> ## Key Concepts: Chapter 8
>
> Legal Issues in Documentation
> Language Application Model for Patient Care Practices

LANGUAGE APPLICATION MODEL FOR PATIENT CARE PRACTICES

Patient care practice is a phrase that encompasses both the goal and execution of nursing. The intent of Chapter 8, examining how documentation affects patient care medically and legally, explained the intricate and necessary role of precise and accurate language to meet this criteria. It introduces a model for language use that demonstrates the interconnected nature of nursing process, documentation, and legal and financial case review.

Chapter 8 explained how each nurse benefits from having a knowledge base that includes the understanding of their state's Nurse Practice Act, government regulations, and to understand the Patient's Bill of Rights. These are not simply legal guidelines. They are tools that enable each nurse to enhance his or her personal level of practice and to fulfill the nurse's primary role as patient care advocate.

As a care advocate the nurse knows that communication is key to appropriate intervention and care. It provides the information necessary for insurance providers, including those disbursing public funds, to justify reimbursement of costs to health care facilities. With health care costs rising it is absolutely necessary to justify care. It may feel like nurses become accountants; however, it only makes sense to be aware that economics play a role in health care. If documentation is inadequate and reimbursement to providers is denied or withheld, patient care is also affected. The good news is that the same language and documentation standards necessary for medical and legal standards will most likely meet the need of the payor. The patient is served, patient care meets the highest standard, and nurses benefit by a job well done. Job satisfaction is beneficial to continued good practice, stable staffing with fewer turnovers, and a healthy medical care environment.

Quality care is a multifaceted goal. It is a goal that is met when nurses understand that each facet of their job contributes to accomplishing the best patient care possible. By approaching nursing with the understanding that details do make a difference, and by appreciating the complexity of the health care industry, nurses are better equipped to provide care and meet the needs of all that is required of them: by their patients, by their employer, by the legal system, and most importantly, by themselves.

SUGGESTIONS FOR CLINICAL SETTINGS

It may be helpful to carry 3 × 5 cards with charting guidelines that you want to reinforce in the clinical setting. We recommend carrying cards that list the divisions of the CHH and H & P. Cards can also be purchased for this purpose. Cards can be secured together by punching a hole in the corner and using a single ring. Medical students use this technique for keeping brief records of their patients. The cards fit in your pocket and are available for quick reference for updating patient information.

Another useful tool is to write down the format preferred for verbal report. It is then a simple matter of "filling in the blanks" with specific patient information from the reference notes on each patient. It is not good practice to report vague patient information. With minimal planning it is possible to have organized data readily available for reporting or documenting purposes.

Figure 9.1
Reference card: symptom characteristics. Add subcategories to help you recall specific questions for your interview.

SYMPTOM CHARACTERISTICS

LOCATION

QUALITY

QUANTITY

CHRONOLOGY ONSET/DURATION

ASSOCIATED MANIFESTATIONS

ALLEVIATING

AGGRAVATING

MEANING TO PATIENT

Figure 9.2
Reference card: reminder of categories of CHH and other critical data.

CHH

ID	***CONCURRENT DX**
PP	***MEDICATIONS**
HPI	***ALLERGIES**
PHX	
FHX	
OCCHX	
P/S HX	
ROS	

Figure 9.3
Reference card: quick reference for recall of patient and critical data.

ID:

CC:

HPI:

PHX:

    MEDS

     ALLERGIES

FHX:

P/S HX:

ROS:

VS:

LABS:

Figure 9.4
Reference card: verbal report and reminder of qualities of good documentation.

VERBAL REPORT

ID, AGE, DX, CC, VS, SX, ASSOC. FACTORS, LABS, INTERVENTIONS, Δ/OUTCOME.

PRIORITIZATION	**BREVITY**
RELEVENCE	**EFFICIENCY**
OBJECTIVE/QUANTITY	**ACCURACY**

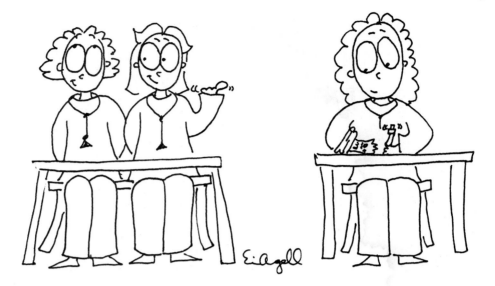

It may also be helpful to bring this book to clinical with you. We find that oral report and written documentation can be stressful simply because the process is unfamiliar. Having a "cheat sheet" to remind the nurse of a specific word or syntax relieves anxiety and allows for more fluid thought. Students often believe that they are expected to return information from memory. This is a fundamentally unsound practice. In the first place, the data need to be correct and memory aids can minimize the risk of error; second, the newness of the situation adds stress to the student who is entering information into the patient record. And, the pressure of "performing" for an instructor and or experienced staff members can be overwhelming and intimidating. The student who feels they have done poorly may feel humiliated and become increasingly timid with verbal report.

Refer to the clinical policy and procedure manual for questions regarding medication and fluid replacement documentation. Note additional information in the narrative when circumstances demand further explanation. Laws that govern nursing practice cannot be superceded by a hospital's policy. Nurse functions that overlap with that of other providers are governed by limited policy or standing orders. Nurses should not feel that a facility's practice of minimal charting with standard forms only excuses them from precise documentation. It does not.

The final note is to emphasize the importance of *prioritization*, *relevancy*, organization, brevity, accuracy, and *efficiency* in reporting and documenting. Use sound concepts and practice, practice, practice. Nurses can improve their own practice standards and improve patient care management.

APPENDIX A

Common Abbreviations

Medicine not only has an technical language of its own it also has many acronyms and specialty abbreviations incorporated into the verbal and written communication. Nurses are responsible for knowing the acceptable abbreviations specific to their workplace. There are many commonly identified abbreviations, although not all are used or accepted at every facility. Be sure to check your facility's policy as to what is approved where you work. Below are some commonly accepted abbreviations. Many may have been used in this workbook.

a	before	BM	bowel movement
abd	abdomen	BP	blood pressure
ac	with meals	BRN	Board of Registered Nursing
A.D.	right ear	BSA	body surface area
A.S.	left ear	BSE	breast self exam
A.U.	both ears	bx.	biopsy
A. Fib	atrial fibrillation	c̄	with
AIDS	acquired immune deficiency syndrome	Ca	cancer
		CABG	coronary artery bypass graft
AK	above the knee	CAD	coronary artery disease
AKA	also known as	CAPD	continuous ambulatory peritoneal dialysis
am	morning		
AMA	against medical advice	CAT	computerized axial tomography
angio	angiogram		
A & O	alert and oriented	cath.	catheter
A-P	anterior-posterior	CBC	complete blood count
AP	apical pulse	cc	cubic centimeter
ARDS	adult respiratory distress syndrome	c/c or C/C	chief complaint
		CCU	coronary care unit; cardiac care unit
ASA	aspirin		
asap	as soon as possible	cert.	certification
ASHD	arteriosclerotic vascular heart disease	chemo	chemotherapy
		CHF	congestive heart failure
AWOL	absent without leave	CNS	central nervous system
B.A.	blood alcohol	con't	continued
BS	breath sounds	c/o	complaints of; complains of
BBS	bilateral breath sounds	COPD	chronic obstructive pulmonary disease
B & C	board and care		
BIB	brought in by	CP	chest pain
bid	twice a day	CSF	cerebral spinal fluid
bilat	bilateral	CVA	cerebral vascular accident
BK	below the knee	d	day

D&C	dilation & curettage	GU	genitourinary
d/c	discontinue	GYN	gynecology
dept.	department	HA	headache
DIC	disseminated intravascular coagulation	HB/Hbg	hemoglobin
disp.	disposition	hct	hematocrit
DM	diabetes mellitus	HCTZ	hydrochlorothiazide
DNR	do not resuscitate	hep A	hepatitis A
D.O.	doctor of osteopathy	hep B	hepatitis B
DOA	dead on arrival	hep C	hepatitis C
DOB	date of birth	HHA	home health aide
DPAHC	durable power of attorney for health care	h/o	history of
		HOB	head of bed
DPT	diphtheria, pertussis, tetanus vaccination	HOH	hard of hearing
		H&P	history & physical
drsg.	dressing	H.R.	heart rate
DSD	dry, sterile dressing	hrs.	hours
DTs	delirium tremors	hs	bedtime
dx	diagnosis	HTN	hypertension
EBL	estimated blood loss	Hx.	history
EKG	electrocardiogram	I&D	incision & drainage
ED	emergency department	ICU	intensive care unit
ER	emergency room	IDDM	insulin dependent diabetes mellitus
EDC	estimated date of confinement	IM	intramuscular
EEG	electroencephalogram	inj.	injection
ENT	ear, nose and throat	I&O	intake & output
ESRF	end stage renal failure	irreg.	irregular
eta	estimated time of arrival	IV	intravenous
ETOH	ethanolism, alcoholism, under an intoxicated state	IVPB	intravenous piggyback
		IVP	intravenous push; intravenous pyelogram
ETT	endotracheal tube	IUD	intrauterine device
eval	evaluate, evaluation	IZ	immunization
exp.	expiratory	JCAHO	Joint Commission on Accreditation of Hospitals
F	female		
FB	foreign body	JVD	jugular vein distention
FBS	fasting blood sugar	K+	potassium
FSBG	finger stick blood glucose	KCl	potassium chloride
FSBS	finger stick blood sugar	kg	kilogram
f/c	Foley catheter	L or Lt.	left
FLB	funny looking beat	LAC	left antecubital
FNP	family nurse practitioner	lac.	laceration
fr.	French	lat.	lateral
frq.	frequent	lb.	pound
fx	fracture	LCSW	licensed clinical social worker
G.B.	gallbladder		
gd.	good	L&D	labor and delivery
GD	gravely disabled	LE	lower extremity
GI	gastrointestinal	LLE	left lower extremity
G#, P#, SAB#, TAB#	Gravida, Para, Spontaneous Abortion, Therapeutic Abortion	LLC	long leg cast
		LLL	left lower lobe
		LLQ	left lower quadrant
glut.	gluteal	LMP	last menstrual period
gm.	gram	LNMP	last normal menstrual period
grav.	gravida		

LOC	level of consciousness	ortho.	orthopedic
LS	lumbosacral	ortho VS	orthopedic vital signs
L. spine	lumbar spine	OS	left eye
LUA	left upper arm	OTC	over the counter
LUE	left upper extremity	OU	both eyes
LUL	left upper lobe	$\bar{p}$	after
LUQ	left upper quadrant	pac	premature atrial contraction
LVN	licensed vocational nurse	PACU	post anesthesia care unit
lytes	electrolytes	palp.	palpation
M	male	PAT	paroxysmal atrial
MAE	moves all extremities		tachycardia
ma. or maj.	major	pc	after meals
max.	maximal	pcn	penicillin
mcg	micrograms	PDR	Physician's Desk Reference
MD	medical doctor	PE	physical examination
mec.	meconium	peds.	pediatrics
med.	medicine	periph.	peripheral
mEq/L	milliequivalent per liter	perc.	percutaneous
mg	milligram	PERLA	pupils equal and reactive to
MgSO4	magnesium sulfate		light and accommodation
MHU	mental health unit	pm	afternoon
MI	myocardial infarction	PMD	private medical doctor
min.	minimum	pneumo.	pneumothorax
ml	milliliter	po	by mouth, oral
mod.	moderate	post-op	postoperative
MRI	magnetic resonance imaging	pr	per rectum
MS	multiple sclerosis or mitral	prn	as needed
	stenosis	pt.	patient
mtg.	meeting	p/w/d	pale, warm, dry
muc.	mucus	q.	each, every
Na.	sodium	q.am	every morning
n/a	not applicable	q.d.	every day
n/c	nasal cannula	q.i.d.	four times per day
NG	nasogastric	q.h.	each hour
neg.	negative	q.h.s.	every night
neuro.	neurological	qs	quantity sufficient
NKA	no known allergies	qns	quantity not sufficient
NKDA	no known drug allergies	quad.	quadriceps
noc.	nocturnal	quan.	quantity
nl.	normal	R or Rt.	right
NPO	nothing by mouth	RAC	right antecubital
NS	normal saline	RLE	right lower extremity
nsg.	nursing	RLL	right lower lobe
NSR	normal sinus rhythm	RLQ	right lower quadrant
n/t	nontender	RUA	right upper arm
NTG	nitroglycerine	RUE	right upper extremity
n/v	nausea and vomiting	RUL	right upper lobe
O2	oxygen	RUQ	right upper quadrant
OB	obstetrical	re:	regarding, about
occas.	occasional	rec'd.	received
OCP	oral contraceptives	reg.	regular
OD	right eye	resp.	respirations or respiratory
OR	operating room	rm.	room
ORIF	open reduction with internal	r/o	rule out
	fixation	ROS	review of systems

rt.	respiratory therapy	TIA	transient ischemic attack
rx.	treatment	tid	three times daily
s̄	without	TKO	to keep open
sat'd.	saturated	tol.	tolerated
syst.	systolic	TPR	temperature, pulse,
sens.	sensation or sensitivity		respiration
sl.	slight	TSE	testicular self-exam
sc.	scant	tx.	traction
SNF	skilled nursing facility	URI	upper respiratory infection
SOAP	subjective, objective,	UTI	urinary tract infection
	assessment, and plan	vag.	vaginal
SOB	shortness of breath	V. Fib.	ventricular fibrillation
sq or subq.	subcutaneous	V. Tach.	ventricular tachycardia
spont.	spontaneous	VNA	Visiting Nurses Association
ST or S. tach.	sinus tachycardia	VS	vital signs
stat	immediately	VSS	vital signs stable
STD	sexually transmitted disease	W&D	warm & dry
sub ling.	sublingual	WNL	within normal limits
SVT	supraventricular tachycardia	w/o	without
sx.	symptoms	wt.	weight
TAB	therapeutic abortion	w/c	wheelchair
TB	tuberculosis	y/o	years old
TCU	transitional care unit or		
	telemetry care unit		

APPENDIX B

Glossary

The following list is by no means comprehensive. It is a collection of interesting words commonly used in both nontechnical and technical communication. A suggested exercise would be to expand upon this list.

abandonment
Common: desertion
Technical: not fulfilling obligation toward patient

accessory
Common: something extra but nonessential; someone who helps another break laws
Technical: auxiliary, as with muscles or nerves

accommodate
Common: willing to do a favor; provide lodging; a convenience
Technical: state of adjustment or adaptation especially eye; focus

advanced
Common: highly developed; complex
Technical: far along in course

alter
Common: change; tailor; castrate or spay
Technical: significant change

amplitude
Common: great size; fullness
Technical: measure of an action potential

anterior
Common: front location
Technical: reference in anatomical position to areas facing forward

appendix
Common: supplemental section at end of book
Technical: an appendage, most commonly related to the small bowel

appreciate
Common: think well of or value
Technical: recognize quality of symptom

arrest
Common: seize and hold under legal authority
Technical: stopped, as in organ function or disease process

articulate
Common: well-spoken
Technical: jointed; surface meeting of joints

artifact
Common: man-made object, often of historical interest
Technical: anything caused incidentally by technique used rather than natural occurrence

atraumatic
Common: no trauma
Technical: without trauma

bag
Common: flexible container; to grab or capture; area of interest
Technical: pouch or container to hold and/or measure body fluids or drainage

beat
Common: hit repeatedly; surpass or defeat
Technical: stroke or pulsation

bed
Common: sleeping furniture; ground for planting
Technical: supporting structure for tissue

bias
Common: diagonal line across grain of fabric; preference that interferes with impartial judgment
Technical: prejudiced or subjective attitude; not objectively represented in a balanced fashion

block
Common: solid section of wood usually with flat sides; section of a city with defined parameters
Technical: interruption in the transmission of impulse, e.g., cardiac or nerve

boring
Common: dull; repetitive
Technical: drilling or digging sensation

calf
Common: baby, young cow
Technical: muscular area of the lower portion of the leg

capture
Common: seize or take possession of by force; represent
Technical: normal response of heart muscle to electrical impulse

character
Common: traits that define a person's integrity or behavior; a shorthand symbol that represents a value of some description; slang that portrays behavior as interesting and singular
Technical: traits that describe in detail a specific complaint or symptom

collateral
Common: corroborating; supporting; indirect
Technical: subsidiary to primary, as with arteries

compensation
Common: reimbursement
Technical: counterbalance; adjustment for a defect

complaint
Common: expressed dissatisfaction; formal legal charge by plaintiff
Technical: ailment, problem or symptom expressed by patient

compliant
Common: yielding
Technical: measure by which an organ deforms or distends adheres to recommended course of treatment

compress
Common: condense
Technical: pads or gauze applied for pressure, heat, or coldness

conduction
Common: transmission
Technical: transmission of energy from one point to another

contraction
Common: shortened word form
Technical: muscle shortening or an increase in tension; heartbeat; expulsive muscle shortening during labor

coping
Common: decorative covering along edges of wall
Technical: ability to face; resolve problem

cretin
Common: dolt or idiot
Technical: individual with stunted physical growth or mental ability

decline
Common: refuse; reject; descend
Technical: refuse; to deteriorate in condition

deficit
Common: shortfall of money; inadequacy
Technical: insufficient; that which is being consumed faster than replaced

deviant
Common: abandoning normal or proscribed behavior; abnormal, sometimes criminal, behavior
Technical: reaction that fails to respond in expected fashion; differing from standard or norm

digit
Common: number
Technical: finger or toe

dilate
Common: enlarge or expand
Technical: enlarge cavity either through intention, disease process, or normal response

discharge
Common: relieve of a burden or task; to fire from a job
Technical: secretion or excretion of a body fluid; release from care

discipline
Common: punishment; training for strict order or behavior
Technical: specific medical specialty

drain
Common: draw off liquid; channel or pipe; to empty
Technical: tube to remove discharge or fluid from cavity

dress
Common: to put on clothes; one-piece style of woman's apparel
Technical: apply cover to support or protect wound

eliminate
Common: get rid of; to remove
Technical: expel waste material from body

elopement
Common: run away to get married
Technical: patient who leaves against medical recommendation or secretly

evacuate
Common: withdraw from a hazardous place; vacate
Technical: empty, especially bowel waste; remove from, as with uterine contents

excitement
Common: easily provoked state; state of high emotion
Technical: degree of potential for stimulation

excursion
Common: short trip or outing usually for pleasure; digression
Technical: deviation from expected normal course

expel
Common: dismiss or drive out
Technical: emit gas or matter from a body cavity

expire
Common: come to an end; to die
Technical: breathe out; to die

exquisite
Common: elaborately done; beautiful
Technical: intense, keen or sharp in character

failure
Common: to fall short or be deficient; unsuccessful
Technical: inability to function; to miss medical appointment

fixation
Common: strong attachment or obsession
Technical: being immobilized and firmly attached; preserving tissue sample for analysis

flush
Common: to flow copiously; to blush or turn red; poker hand with cards all in the same suit; hunting term for exposing game birds; to wash out a toilet with copious amounts of water
Technical: to irrigate or wash out with large amounts of water; skin condition secondary to capillary dilation

force
Common: strength or power; compel or inflict against resistance; large group
Technical: to introduce food through tube to one unwilling or unable to eat

hardware
Common: articles made of metal; tools; parts of a computer
Technical: orthopedic appliances for internal or external use

humor
Common: ability to be funny, comic
Technical: fluid or semifluid substance in body

illness
Common: sickness
Technical: abnormal process that interrupts or diminishes a person's functioning

impaired
Common: diminished; harmed
Technical: weakened; damaged; deteriorated

implant
Common: to set firmly; instill
Technical: graft; insert in tissue; put in surgically

incompetence
Common: a lack of ability
Technical: organs which are not functioning properly

incompetent
Common: not qualified
Technical: organs that are not functioning properly; person legally proclaimed unable to manage his or her own affairs

incontinent
Common: not controlled; unable to be restrained
Technical: unable to control excretory functions

indolent
Common: lazy
Technical: not active; not an active medical problem

injection
Common: forcing of one element (gas or liquid) into another (ground); introducing a subject into a discussion
Technical: introducing medicine into tissue or vein; congestion or hyperemia, as with a red eye

injury
Common: wound or damage; injustice
Technical: any environmental interruption in a person's ability to adapt or defend state of well-being

insipid
Common: dull; without flavor or tasteless
Technical: not arousing interest; vague

insult
Common: derogatory reference to another or to self
Technical: break in integrity; traumatic event

intake
Common: a taking in; place in a pipe where water is taken in
Technical: amount of food or fluid absorbed by patient

integrity
Common: honesty; strictness of values
Technical: soundness of structure; unimpaired status

intolerance
Common: unbearable nature; bigotry
Technical: inability to handle substance or inability to endure

intervention
Common: coming between or interference
Technical: action to alter or modify a process

invasive
Common: denoting an act of violating; tending to overrun harmfully
Technical: denoting a puncture, incision, or penetration of the body; relating to the spread of neoplasm to adjoining tissue

irreversible
Common: impossible to reverse
Technical: condition that cannot be turned back

irrigation
Common: to water, artificially
Technical: to wash wound with saline or medicated fluids

labor
Common: work or task; those who do work for others for wages
Technical: effort expended for activity as breathing; process of delivering fetus

lacerate
Common: rip or tear
Technical: tear tissue; wound with jagged edge

lacrimation
Common: related to tears
Technical: tears

lactate
Common: to secrete milk
Technical: a product of lactic acid; to produce milk

lead
Common: to guide or direct; to be at head; dull gray metal
Technical: connection for electrical conduction usually between a patient and measuring device

line
Common: narrow continuous mark; boundary; covering for an interior surface
Technical: access cannula for vascular testing or medicating

local
Common: person from a particular area; branch of labor union
Technical: not general or systemic; anesthetic limited to one area

loose
Common: not tightly fastened, bound, stapled, or bundled; not exact in interpretation; demonstrating lack of restraint; immoral
Technical: not formed or bound together in reference to stool or tissue; mental associations implying disordered thought process

macerate
Common: to soak in liquid to soften and separate into components
Technical: to soften or make thin

main
Common: most important; large pipe or conduit
Technical: primary source, such as coronary arteries

maintain
Common: to continue; to keep in good condition
Technical: to comply with good health practice

mass
Common: nonspecific quantity or amount of matter; reference to greatest number of members of common group; religious celebration
Technical: number of cells grouped together, such as tumor; physical properties of matter that give it measurable dimensions

met
Common: past tense of the word *meet*
Technical: shortened form of the word *metastasis* (spread or implant of neoplasm to other tissue)

mole
Common: small mammal; undercover spy
Technical: small, raised growth on skin; intrauterine mass

morbid
Common: gruesome, grisly; unwholesome preoccupation
Technical: related to disease; deviant

moribund
Common: near death
Technical: dying; death imminent

murmur
Common: low continuous sound; mutter
Technical: soft sound heard while listening to heart or vessels

needleless
Common: no needle
Technical: any system which has been modified to eliminate needle use

noncompliant
Common: not malleable
Technical: not able or willing to comply with treatment regimen

nonresponsive
Common: to not reply or to not react
Technical: no reaction, physical or mental, to applied stimulus

obese
Common: extremely overweight
Technical: abnormally overweight by a defined percentage.

objective
Common: material rather than mental concept; uninfluenced by personal feelings
Technical: clinical sign that can be seen, heard or measured; goal; lens of microscope

obtunded
Common: oblivious to external stimuli
Technical: reduced level of consciousness due to analgesia, or use of drugs or alcohol

ordinary
Common: usual; not exceptional
Technical: within a standard, expected performance standards

output
Common: amount of work, energy, or product produced within a time frame
Technical: quantity of urine, excretion, or other measured substance over a given period

papoose
Common: Native American infant
Technical: method for restraining a child for a procedure

patent
Common: government document that ensures inventor's rights; the obvious
Technical: opened, not plugged

pattern
Common: design or model; routine way of doing things
Technical: recognizable model; repetitive behavior trait

persistent
Common: enduring; continuing firmly in spite of obstacle
Technical: obstinate continuation, despite the environmental conditions

phalanx
Common: a tightly grouped formation
Technical: singular for long bones of fingers

piggyback
Common: term for one person carrying another on shoulders; truck trailer carried on the flat car of train
Technical: to deliver a bag of IV solution by injecting into existing IV tubing

potential
Common: latent; expected capacity for development
Technical: possible but not real; action which may take place under proscribed conditions

pounding
Common: striking repeatedly; crushing by forceful beating
Technical: heavy throbbing sensation

quadrant
Common: altitude determining instrument; mathematical plane
Technical: division of an anatomical region for purpose of description

radiation
Common: emission of rays; glowing manifestation
Technical: to spread from a focal area

rebound
Common: bounce or spring back; recover after a let down
Technical: sudden contraction of muscle after relaxation; sudden response to an activity or treatment after a stimulus has been removed

reduce
Common: lessen or diminish
Technical: restore by manipulation or surgery to normal position

refuse
Common: declined to accept or allow; discarded as worthless
Technical: decline to do or allow

relief
Common: a lessening of discomfort; aid given to needy; art or map with elevated components
Technical: alleviation of symptom; area under prosthesis intended to reduce pressure

retention
Common: hold; keep possession of; to hire
Technical: keeping body waste, as with urine

reversible
Common: turned backward in position, order, or direction
Technical: turning in opposite direction of disease, symptom, or state

ribbon
Common: narrow strip of cloth or decorative fabric
Technical: stool formed flat and narrow

run
Common: to move rapidly on foot; to compete for an elected office; to drive or steer
Technical: to deliver fluids or medications through IV

scope
Common: the range of action or thought
Technical: instrument for viewing or listening; a range that sets practice parameters

standing
Common: positioned upright
Technical: prepared instructions to be performed automatically under specific conditions

status
Common: legal definition of state of person or thing; high social regard
Technical: condition; assessment of patient state

stool
Common: seat with no back or arms; footrest
Technical: fecal material

stream
Common: body of water running in channel of earth's surface
Technical: steady flow of liquid, especially urine

subjective
Common: personal
Technical: symptom, sensation or assessment that cannot be measured quantitatively

thready
Common: having to do with fibrous strands twisted together; like the ridges on screws or bolts; common element that is cohesive
Technical: description of pulse quality that is weak and rapid, often indicating shock

titrate
Common: determine solution concentration
Technical: deliver solution in a specific concentration over a defined time period

transpose
Common: to change or reverse the order of
Technical: to replace existing IV fluid bag with a new or different bag; to change placement of organs or tissue

trauma
Common: wound
Technical: wound or shock; injury accidental or purposefully inflicted

tremors
Common: trembling as in slight earth shaking
Technical: body movement that is involuntary, usually a slight tremble can be regular or intermittent

trigger
Common: a release for discharging a firearm
Technical: a stimulus for a physiological or chemical event

tube
Common: pipe; hollow cylinder
Technical: canal; hollow organ; any pipe through which oxygen, medication, or food is given, or fluid drained from body orifice

turn
Common: move or cause to move
Technical: change patient position on a regular schedule

valve
Common: structure which regulates the flow of gas or liquid
Technical: membrane of canal or hollow organ that prevents reflux of fluid

vapid
Common: not interested; not lively
Technical: dull, listless

vapors
Common: gaseous state of a normally liquid or solid matter; old-fashioned term for feeling poorly
Technical: inhaled medication

vegetative
Common: relating to plants or plant growth; capable of growth
Technical: not active; growing or functioning involuntarily or unconsciously

void
Common: empty; unoccupied
Technical: to urinate or defecate

APPENDIX C

Computer Application User Guide

The WorkBook program is the computer adjunct for the textbook, *Documentation: The Language of Nursing.* If you are familiar with the Microsoft Windows environment, you can probably install the application and begin using it now. If you are not comfortable with personal computers, you may find the following material beneficial.

INSTALLATION

Insert the CD or floppy disk into your computer, and open File Manager (Windows 3.1) or Explorer (Windows 95 and 98). In the left pane of your screen, double click the left mouse button over the CD-ROM icon, or over the floppy drive icon if you have the floppy version. Find the "Install" file or "Install.exe" file in the right pane of your screen, and double click the left mouse on this file's icon. This will start the Installation program. From here, just follow the prompts provided. It is suggested that you accept the Installer's recommendations unless you are sure of what you are doing. If this installation procedure made no sense to you, read the next section, "Basic Usage," and then come back to this installation section.

BASIC USAGE

The mouse is a pointing device used to move a cursor around your computer screen. Moving the mouse moves the cursor. Pressing the button on the left side of the mouse generally initiates an action when the cursor is over certain symbols on the screen. This is called "clicking." Generally, these symbols look like push buttons, or are colored, underlined text. Sometimes, the shape of the cursor will change in some way to indicate to you that a click of the left mouse button can initiate an action, but this isn't always the case.

The mouse is also used to scroll areas of the screen up, down, left, and right. These screen areas are usually called "windows." Scrollbars indicate the area of a window used to accomplish scrolling. The ends of each scrollbar show direction arrows, with an unmarked box between them.

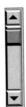 This is what a vertical scrollbar looks like.

Clicking on a direction arrow will cause the window to scroll up or down if it is a vertical scrollbar, or left or right if it is a horizontal scrollbar. Scrolling can also be done by pointing at the unmarked box between the direction arrows and moving the mouse while keeping the left button depressed, in other words, *dragging* the box. Of note, not all windows have scrollbars. This means that all the contents of the window are already visible on your screen.

THE WORKBOOK APPLICATION

The WorkBook Interactive Computer Application requires the use of a mouse. If you are unfamiliar with how a mouse works in the Microsoft Windows environment, please review the preceding section, "Basic Usage."

In the WorkBook Application, the mouse cursor is a small arrow on the screen that moves when you slide the mouse on a mouse pad or other working surface. When the arrow is over a word or area of the window that is interactive, the arrow will change to a pointing finger. This alerts you that pressing the left mouse button will produce an interactive event. Pressing the left mouse button is called clicking. The type of interaction depends on what kind of window the cursor is in, or the type of exercise being presented.

Generally, getting around the WorkBook, called *navigating,* is accomplished via the push button icons at the top of the screen, or through the Contents window. The navigating buttons provide different actions depending on what is displayed on your screen. Their functions are explained throughout this appendix. While using the WorkBook application, hint text is displayed at the bottom of the screen when the mouse cursor is over one of these buttons. This hint text is a reminder of the function that navigational button provides. Of note, if the text in one of these buttons is gray, that button's function is not available at that time.

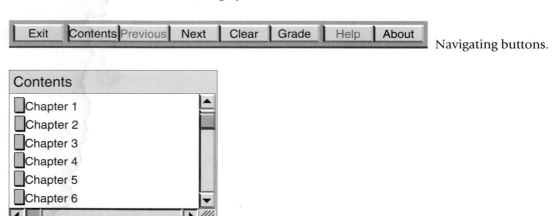

Navigating buttons.

The Contents window provides a central place for accessing any exercise for any chapter. The mouse cursor changes from an arrow to a pointing finger when moved over a chapter. Clicking the left mouse button at this time opens that chapter's contents. To view a list of that chapter's exercises, click on *Exercises.* To view a short summary of the textbook's associated chapter, click *Synopsis.* To work on a specific exercise, click on it; an Answer List window and Exercise Answer Page window will replace the Contents window on the screen. To return to the Contents window, click the "Contents" button at the top of the screen, or click the underlined, blue text "Go to Contents" that is at the bottom of every Exercise Answer Page. Note the vertical scrollbar on the right side of the Contents window. When chapter lists are long, use the scrollbar to scroll the desired list into view.

To begin working *on* exercises, open one as described in the preceding paragraph. Each exercise has an Exercise Answer Page window on the left side of the screen, and an Answer List window on the right. If the mouse cursor is in an Answer List window, it will change to the pointing finger when over a word, and to an outline around a grabbing hand icon when the left mouse button is pressed. This means that word can be *dragged* to an Answer Slot, one of the gray boxes in the Exercise Answer Page window, and *dropped* into that slot by releasing the left mouse button. This is called *drag and drop*. The selected word continues to be part of the Answer List. The drag and drop feature merely copies the word into the Answer Slot. To change an answer, simply drag and drop another word from the Answer List. No deleting is necessary. Clicking the "Clear" button at the top of the screen removes all answers from the Answer Slots.

Answer Slots are the gray boxes in Exercise Answer Page windows. If the box is without an outline, it will accept answers dragged from the Answer List window. You may click on the Answer Slot to view the correct answer. It will appear in a smaller, separate window on your screen. When you have viewed the answer and want to continue, simply click on the OK button in this small window. The answer window will disappear and you may continue working in the exercise.

Some Answer Slots have an *outline* around the gray box. This indicates that the exercise is of a different type than drag and drop. These outlined slots *will not* accept drag and drop words from the Answer List. In fact, there will be no words in the Answer List to grab. Instead, there will be sentences above the outlined Answer Slot with Hot Text. Hot Text are merely words that, when clicked, become part of an answer in an Answer Slot. The mouse cursor changes to a pointing finger when moved over Hot Text. Hot Text turns white with a blue background when clicked, as well as appearing in the Answer Slot below it. To deselect Hot Text, simply click on it again.

There are several ways to get around in the WorkBook application. As already described, the Contents window provides access to every exercise. Once in an Exercise Answer Page, you can also move back and forth from one exercise to another by clicking the "Previous" and "Next" buttons at the top of the screen, or the underlined blue text "Go to Next" or "Go to Previous" at the bottom of the Exercise Answer Page.

Depending on the type of exercise, there are several ways to check your answers. Clicking on any gray Answer Slot displays a message box with your answer, the correct answer, and associated information regarding that specific question. Clicking the "Grade" button at the top of the screen displays an Exercise Graded Answers window, which shows your answers, the correct answers, and grading results, for the entire exercise.

Every exercise provides specific instructions at the top of the Exercise Answer Page. Exercise 1.1 is a demonstration exercise, providing an explanation for each exercise type you may encounter in the WorkBook. It is a good place to start.

The WorkBook application also provides a Help screen to remind you of how things work. Click the "Help" button to access this screen.

Index

A

Abbreviations
  common, 238
  exercise in, 51, 62
  institutional, 3, 22, 26b, 216
  standardized, 3
Accuracy, 219–220, 237
Action, language that implies, 82–84,
    88–89, 222
Active listening, 95
Adjectives
  limitation of, 102
  vs. descriptors, 3
Advocacy, 194, 194b, 233
Age, in patient profile, 43, 43b
Alleviating/aggravating factors, 141b,
    141–142
  identification exercise for, 142–143, 150
  in response to symptoms, 141b,
    141–142
Appearance, of patient, 121b
Arrows, meaning of, 22–23
Assessment data
  purpose of, 196–197
  word selection for, 196–197
Assignment despite objection, 190b
Associated manifestations
  description of, 139b
  exercises in, 139–141, 150
  overlap with timing and setting, 139
Assumptions, 102

B

Bias
  effects of, 97–98
  patient sources of, 97–99
  from personal experience, 99
  politically correct attitude *vs.*, 98b
  self-knowledge of, 95
Bias words, 94
  sources of, 223
Brevity, 220, 222, 237

C

Change, symbol for, 22, 22f
Charting
  of actual and potential problems,
    78–81
  case studies in, 74–75
  descriptive data in, 69

essence of, 76, 88
exceptional, 2
exercise in, 76, 88
format in, 75–76
handwriting in, 18–19, 19f, 20f
problem-oriented, 40–41, 41b
samples of, 206–215
simple, 74–77, 76f
spelling in, 17–18
Checklists, 93
  in charting, 2
  vs. narrative charting, 220
CHH. *See* Complete health history
    (CHH)
Chief complaint
  in complete health history, 40–41
  exercise for, 46, 61
  patient evaluation of, 94
  in patient profile, 45–46
  in SOAP format, 46b
  in symptom interview, 120–121
Chronology
  case study example of, 136
  descriptor matching exercise in,
    136–137, 150
  descriptors used in, 134b
  relationship exercise in, 135–136, 150
  as timing of symptom, 134b, 134–135
Clinical pathways, 77b
  objective goals in, 227
Clinical settings
  charting suggestions for, 234, 235f,
    236f
  hospital policy and procedure manual
    in, 237
Colloquialisms, use of, 104
Common terms
  technical meaning exercise with, 8–9,
    32
  technical meanings of, 6–7
  unfamiliar definitions of, 8–9
Competence, standard of, 194b
Complaint. *See* Chief complaint
Complete health history (CHH), 40–42,
    40–58, 59b
  "by the way" information in, 54b
  concurrent health problems in, 47–48
  family history in, 50, 52b
  first impressions in, 48b
  head to toe format of, 55
  history of present illness in, 47, 47b

informant in, 42, 42b
occupational/environmental history
    in, 51, 52b
past health history in, 48–50,
    50b–51b
patient profile in, 42–44
personal/social history in, 52, 53b
pertinent details in, 49b
problem list in, 55, 56b
problem-oriented, 40–41, 41b
reference card for, 234f
review of systems in, 52–53, 54b
samples of, 59b, 63–66
status post, 55–56
as sytem of organization, 41–42
Completeness, 202, 204
Consistency, 203–204
  in charting, 186, 191
  in documentation, 1
  in format, 2, 219–220
  in language use, 2
  in measurement, 104–105, 105b
  in measurement definitions, 104–105
  in objective measurements, 227
  in verbal report, 1
Context
  actual and potential problems in,
    78–81
  word meaning in, 8–9, 32
Control, patient need for, 111
Cost recovery, and documentation, 189
Critical thinking, language and, 3–4
Culture
  in patient profile, 43
  perception of symptoms and, 94

D

Data
  integration of, 221–222
  subjective *vs.* objective, 93–94
Decrease, symbol for, 23, 23f
Defensible documentation, 187–188
  language requirements for, 188
  patient care standards in, 188
  samples and legal issues, 206–215
Degrees of motion, symbol for, 29, 29f
Description, degrees of, 113b
Descriptors, 73–74
  adjectives *vs.*, 3
  for assessment data, 196–197
  for assessment note, 220

Descriptors, (*continued*)
　for chronology, 134b
　for difficult patients, 111
　of location, 120, 123b–124b, 125,
　　127, 149
　in review of systems, 120, 123b, 125,
　　127
　syntax and, 221
Diagrams, for lab values, 26, 26f
Difficult patients
　descriptors for, 111
　objectivity *vs.* subjectivity with, 111
Documentation
　abbreviations in, 3, 22, 26b
　format of, 40
　inclusive, 2
　medical-legal consequences of, 2, 3
　of patient interview, 29–30
　symbols in, 22–29
　tools for, 93
Documentation standards, JCAHO iden-
　tification of, 188
Drawing conclusions, in documentation,
　198b

E

Economic class, bias and, 99
Efficiency, 2, 220, 222, 237
Electronic charting, 193, 217
Emotion, negative words and, 103
Emphasis, on word and meaning,
　12–13, 33
Employment status, in patient profile, 43
Error
　avoidance of, 189, 190b, 191
　correction of, 189, 190b, 191
Exceptional charting, defined, 2
Expertise, with time and practice, 109,
　227
Expert witness testimony, on patient care
　and standards of practice, 185b

F

Factual data
　in charting and notes, 103
　in conclusions, 103
　in nursing diagnoses, 103
Familiar words, common use meaning
　vs. technical meaning of, 6–7
Family, in evaluation of patient response
　to illness, 96b
Family history, in complete health his-
　tory, 50, 52b
First impressions, in complete health
　history, 48b
Food poisoning, 137
Forensic charting, 199b
Format. *See also* Complete health history
　(CHH); SOAP
　benefit of, 69–70
　in charting, 75
　consistency of, 219–220
　in documentation, 3, 40
　sequential, ordered, 200–201

G

Gender, in patient profile, 43
General appearance, 121b
Goals
　objectification of, 226
　objective parameters for, 110–111
　reimbursement and, 228
Greater than symbol, 27f, 27–28

H

Handwriting
　in charting, 18–19
　legibility of, 198, 200
　　impact on patient care, 219
　samples of poor and illegible, 19f, 20f
Head to toe format, 55, 220, 222
Health care, as personal to patient, 111
Health habits, bias and, 98
Hunches, 112–114
　basis of, 113
　patient support of, 114
　in verbal report, 114
Hygiene, bias and, 99

I

Incident reports, objectivity in, 189, 191
Increase, symbol for, 22, 22f
Individual responsibility, 188–189
Inflammatory words, 100–101, 117,
　224–225
Informed consent
　patient understanding in, 225
　requirements for, 195, 195b
Initial observation, 70
Institutional language standard, 218
Institutional policies and procedures
　in charting, 194, 196
Instruction
　correction and adaptation in, 10
　Socratic technique in, 81
　technical language in, 9–10
Integration, of theoretical and functional
　knowledge, 81–82
Interpretation, *vs.* objective report, 106
Intervention, integration of knowledge
　for, 81–82
Intuitive data, 112–114, 228

J

Journals, views of, 195b
Judgment statements, 100–101, 106b,
　117, 224–225

K

Knowledge, integration of theoretical
　and functional, 81–82

L

Lab values, diagrams for, 26, 26f
Language
　actionable, 82–84, 88–99
　in clinical practice, 69–70
　efficient use of, 2
　impact on patient care, 21
　learning of, 9–10
Language applications model for nurse
　practice, 191f
　language use standards in, 198–201
　legal review in, 233–234
　legal review standards in, 202–204
　quality of care in, 234
　quality of care requirements in,
　　193–198
　reimbursement requirements and, 204
　reimbursement review in, 233–234
　in sample charting, 206–215
Language skills
　critical thinking and, 3–4
　nursing application of, 15–16
Language standards in documentation,
　198–201

forensic charting and, 199b
legibility, 198, 200
objectivity, 201
sequential, ordered format in,
　200–201
spelling, 198, 200, 200b
word picture in, 201b
Learning the language, 218
　memorization in, 14
Legal issues, 185–187
　defensible documentation samples
　　and, 206–215
　informed consent, 195, 195b
　quality of care and, 194–195
　standards of practice and, 185
Legal record of care
　factual *vs.* subjective data in, 103
　objective statements in, 13–14
Legal review
　language pitfalls and, 187b
　standards of care and, 191
Legal standard of practice, 185
　technical terms and, 11–12
Legal standards of review
　charting for patient events, care, case
　　review, 202
　completeness and, 202, 204
　consistency and, 203–204
　documentation language for, 202–204
　systems format for, 202
Less than symbol, 27f, 27–28
Location, of symptoms, 120,
　123b–124b, 125, 126f, 127

M

Malpractice, 201, 202
Marital status, in patient profile, 43
Meaning, standardizing of, 1–4
Meaning of symptom to patient,
　143b–144b
　as aspect of complaint, 143
　body language and, 144b
　case study of, 145
　factors influencing, 143b
　key words in, 144b
Measurement
　common techniques for, 105b
　consistent definition of, 104–105
　within established parameters, 105
Medical-legal concerns
　documentation and, 1, 2, 3
　standards of practive and, 184
　technical terms and, 11–12
Medicare, documentation requirements
　for, 188

N

NANDA. *See* North American Nursing
　Diagnosis Association (NANDA)
Narrative charting, 218
　case study exercise in, 145–146
　key concepts in, 220
　nurse's use of, 192
Negative symbol, 23, 24f
Negative words, sample, 103b
Negligence, 202, 203
Normal
　documented finding matching exer-
　　cise, 109, 117
　individual differences in, 107–108
　vs. abnormal, 227
Normally abnormal patient, charting for,
　227